Healing
with the
Chakra
Energy System

Healing
with the
Chakra
Energy System

ACUPRESSURE, BODYWORK,
AND REFLEXOLOGY FOR
TOTAL HEALTH

John R. Cross

FCSP, Dr. Ac., MRSH, SRP

Foreword by **Robert A. Charman**, FCSP, MCSP, DipTP

North Atlantic Books
Berkeley, California

Published by North Atlantic Books   Cover design by Susan Quasha
P.O. Box 12327, Berkeley, California 94712   Book design by Brad Greene

Permissions
Figure 2.3 (Associations of the Major Chakras with the Autonomic Nervous System) reproduced by Donald and Pam Budge of Croft Studio from *Gray's Anatomy,* 34th edition, by Henry Gray, edited by D.V. Davies, MA, FRCS, copyright © 1967 by Longmans, Green and Co., Ltd. Used by permission from Lippincott Williams and Wilkins.

Color Plates—Clairvoyant's Views of Chakras
The author sent numerous requests for permission to Quest Books, but did not receive a response. If you have any information, please contact North Atlantic Books.

Printed in the United States of America

Healing with the Chakra Energy System: Acupressure, Bodywork, and Reflexology for Total Health is sponsored by the Society for the Study of Native Arts and Sciences, a nonprofit educational corporation whose goals are to develop an educational and crosscultural perspective linking various scientific, social, and artistic fields; to nurture a holistic view of arts, sciences, humanities, and healing; and to publish and distribute literature on the relationship of mind, body, and nature.

North Atlantic Books' publications are available through most bookstores. For further information, call 800-337-2665 or visit our website at www.northatlanticbooks.com.

Substantial discounts on bulk quantities are available to corporations, professional associations, and other organizations. For details and discount information, contact our special sales department.

Library of Congress Cataloging-in-Publication Data
Cross, John R., Dr.
    Healing with the chakra energy system : acupressure, bodywork, and reflexology for total health / by John R. Cross.
         p. ; cm.
    Includes bibliographical references.
    Summary: "A physiotherapist and acupuncturist describes the complex energy centers of the chakras in detail as a therapeutic discipline and shows how they can be used with acupressure, bodywork, reflexology, cranio-sacral therapy, massage therapy, and healing"—Provided by publisher.
    ISBN-13: 978-1-55643-625-3
    ISBN-10: 1-55643-625-4
    1. Mental healing. 2. Chakras. 3. Acupuncture. I. Title.
    [DNLM: 1. Acupressure—methods. 2. Massage—methods. 3. Medicine, Oriental Traditional. 4. Mind-Body and Relaxation Techniques. WB 369.5.A17 C951h 2006]
    RZ401.C76 2006
    615.8'51—dc22
                                                                    2006014914
                                                                    CIP

1 2 3 4 5 6 7 8 9 DATA 12 11 10 09 08 07 06

CONTENTS

CHAPTER FIVE

Healing ... 243

LIST of FIGURES AND TABLES

COLOR INSERT

THE CLAIRVOYANT'S VIEW OF THE CHAKRAS

FOREWORD

I am delighted to welcome *Healing with the Chakra Energy System: Acupressure, Reflexology, and Healing for Total Health* as the third volume in a series of clinical textbooks written by Dr. John Cross. It follows *Acupressure: Clinical Applications in Musculo-Skeletal Conditions* (2000) and *Acupressure and Reflextherapy in the Treatment of Medical Conditions* (2001). I am pleased to say that a fourth volume discussing the Chakra Energy System and Acupuncture is already in preparation, as are others on Light Touch Reflextherapy and the Holistic Spine.

During his long and distinguished clinical career as a chartered physiotherapist, which has encompassed treating everything from the acute injuries of sports medicine to the most chronic and intractable conditions, Dr. Cross has combined his deep knowledge of anatomy and physiology with his pioneering exploration of Eastern concepts of living energy systems to create a truly holistic approach to physical therapy. For any physiotherapist who wishes to extend his or her understanding of energy medicine within the practice of physiotherapy, this book, written by a colleague whose clinical feet are as firmly planted on the ground as their own, will prove an excellent source. For complementary therapists, it offers an invaluable guide to the clinical discipline of relating bodily symptoms to their causes in body and mind dysfunction.

In the first two chapters, through a concise union of text and illustration that continues throughout the book, Dr. Cross takes the reader through the initially unfamiliar landscape of aura fields and the subtle energy flows through acupoints and meridian networks to their source in the seven major chakras that power the whole: the *élan vital* of life itself. With meticulous attention to detail, Dr. Cross links each energy system with the glands, hormones, nervous system, musculoskeletal structures, skin, and the respiratory, visceral, and reproductive organs and systems of conventional anatomy and physiology. He shows how the ceaseless interaction between body, mind, and spirit and how dysfunction in one, or more than one, of its parts affects the whole. This deep understanding forms the theoretical and clinical foundation for the next three chapters, in which these concepts are translated into diagnosis and practical therapy, often illustrated by case histories, through the disciplines of acupressure and bodywork, reflexology, and healing. These three chapters present the reader with such an astonishingly full exposition of the therapy under review that each is worth the price of the book alone.

For those whose thinking is bounded by the paradigm of Western medicine, the concepts under discussion may seem, at first reading, too "way out" to be assimilated into their clinical practice. I suggest, however, that the case histories in Chapters 3 and 5 should give pause for reflective thought, along with Dr. Cross's in-depth discussion of the "listening posts" of heel and vault of head, which are so crucially important in clinical understanding.

With these "listening posts" in mind I would like to offer an analogy. You are shown a colored pattern that looks rather like a wallpaper frieze and are told that if you look at it in the right way you will see a butterfly in a field of flowers. You try and you try, methodically scanning and analyzing the pattern, with no success. To your increasing frustration it remains a pattern with no butterfly and no flowers in sight. After a while your tired mind starts to relax, and you cease all that active mental doing. Your eyes lose their sharp focus, and suddenly, to your astonishment, the two-dimensional frieze dissolves away to reveal a three-dimensional picture of a butterfly poised in a field of flowers. It was there all the time, a 3-D picture hidden in the 2-D pattern, a hidden reality that could only reveal itself when your noisy mind relaxed into quiet receptivity. The inner reality of your patient's being is as important as the outer reality of clinical symptoms in which it is cloaked. What Dr. Cross is getting across in this book is that your patient exists in more than one dimension of reality, and that each dimension has something to tell you. Of course you must take a case history. Of course you must perform a clinical examination, and of course you must take notes, but, and this is a very important *but*, at some point you must stop all this busy "doing." You must be still. You must, in effect, just "be," and in that state of "being" you must "listen" to what the patient's body, mind, and spirit are trying to whisper to you in a language you will only understand if you allow yourself to tune in. As this inner picture reveals itself, your choice of gentle therapy then becomes a healing, in the true sense of the word, into wholeness.

As I was writing this foreword I received news that Dr. Cross has been made a Fellow of the Chartered Society of Physiotherapy, in full recognition of the path he has blazed in integrating Eastern concepts with Western physiotherapy practice. No one has done more to advance this important aspect of physiotherapy theory and practice. I am sure that all those he has inspired, and continues to inspire, through his writings, lectures, seminars, and workshops will feel that the Society's award of FCSP is a well-deserved tribute to his high professional standards and achievements.

Robert A. Charman, FCSP, MCSP, DipTP

Spring 2006

Robert Charman is the editor of *Complementary Therapies for Physical Therapists* (Butterworth Heinemann, 2000). He is also the founder chairman of the Association of Chartered Physiotherapists in Energy Medicine and the chair of the Confederation of Healing Organizations.

INTRODUCTION

I am often asked how I became interested in chakras and what possessed me to spend so many years of my professional life in their study. I started to be interested in the topic in 1968 after my engagement to Andrea. Her father, Fred, was a Spiritualist, and he occasionally took me along to church services to witness those engaged in clairvoyance and healing. He was also a member of an international organization that carried out research in psychical studies. I was more fascinated with the literature sent to him about subtle energy, chakras, and healing than I was in the subject of Spiritualism. In fact, I was a very traditional Christian and later, in the 1980s, became a Methodist Local Preacher. Although Fred was a very learned and important man in the city of London (he was the Master of London Bridge), he was very down-to-earth and not at all what might be considered "way out." This was the main quality I admired and respected about him. Fred was attempting to look at Spiritualism and esoteric matters in a very matter-of-fact manner. One of my favorite teaching expressions is "We can have our heads in the clouds when exploring these phenomena, but we must have our feet on the ground."

In 1970 two momentous events took place: I married Andrea (we are still married after thirty-six years), and I qualified as a chartered and state-registered physical therapist. Initially I was quite happy to ply my trade in general physical therapy, but I soon became aware that I could offer my patients many treatments that weren't necessarily "orthodox." I wanted to *heal* my patients and not just palliate their symptoms, as is so often done in the treatment of chronic medical conditions. I initially studied homeopathy, then radionics, acupuncture, and reflexology in depth. As my awareness of and interest in Chinese Medicine increased, it seemed quite natural to combine this with traditional hands-on therapy. I therefore studied and performed every type of acupressure, shiatsu, and other subtle energy physical medicine approach. It was at this time that my interest in the chakras as important and powerful energy centers in healing, yoga, and meditation was rekindled. I began to wonder whether it would also be possible to use them in physical therapy.

In the mid-1970s there was no literature at all about the Western concept of the chakras as used in therapy and healing. I began to research the subject in depth and to write articles and give talks. I got some very mixed reactions in the early days, especially when lecturing at annual congresses of the Chartered Society of Physiotherapy (CSP) and with the various clinical interest groups. Slowly but surely, though, over the years the techniques of healing with subtle energy have gained more respect. The healing methods that I have created, based on traditional medicine, have been successfully used on thousands of patients. I have also taught these methods to hundreds, if not thousands, of delegates over the past twenty-five years. It has been an enormous privilege to teach this "weird" type of physical medicine. Occasionally I meet some therapists who cannot accept it and who continue to practice what is most comfortable for them. The vast majority of students, however, have accepted the theory and techniques of this art form, and in many cases it has transformed their practices.

I have been asked by countless people to write a book on the chakras. Although I could easily have written it ten or fifteen years ago, perhaps it would not have been accepted as readily as it will be today. It was also important to write my other books—one on acupressure and one on reflextherapy—first, so as to indoctrinate practitioners into a different type of contact healing therapy. I had first introduced the idea of healing with the chakra energy system in a chapter in the book *Complementary Therapies for Physical Therapists* (2000). Using acupressure along with traditional medicine is a forerunner of using acupressure with the chakras. Much more, though, can be achieved with the chakras, since they are far more powerful. I wrote this book specifically for medical therapists in an attempt to make this very versatile and powerful therapy more accessible to the millions of patients worldwide who would benefit from it. Over the past twenty-five years, I have attempted to demystify the chakras and to explain esoteric medicine in as down-to-earth way as possible. I hope therefore to take a leaf out of my late father-in-law's book.

Finally, it is my earnest desire that therapists and practitioners of all persuasions will accept the contents of this book and that the techniques featured here will one day become the therapy of the here and now instead of the future.

This book is dedicated to the memory of Frederick Samuel Hall, with grateful thanks.

CHAPTER ONE

The Subtle Bodies

The number seven is prominent in many aspects of both Western and Eastern philosophy:

- The Earth was created in seven days, or more literally, in seven ages or eras.
- There are seven days in a week.
- There are seven times four days in a lunar month.
- There are seven musical notes in a scale.
- There are seven colors in the spectrum.
- There are said to be seven ages of humankind.
- The Bible refers to the life span as being seventy (seven time ten) years.
- There are seven layers of the skin.
- The physical body is said to change and reproduce itself every seven years.
- There are seven endocrine glands.
- There are seven major spiritual centers, or chakras, which are the seed from which the seven dense and subtle bodies spring.
- There are twenty-one (seven times three) minor chakras.
- There are seven hundred (seven times one hundred) acupuncture and major reflex points.

I could probably think of several more actual and contrived examples. Eastern philosophy talks about the seven heavens, or layers of existence, following the death of the physical body. It is said that the Buddha was transported to nirvana (seventh heaven) during meditation while on the earth plane. The number seven in mentioned in the Bible scores of times. It is mentioned in the book of Revelation (written by St. John the Divine at Patmos) no fewer than on thirty-four occasions, including several references to the seven spirits that man (and of course woman) possesses. It is also a sacred number in Judaism, indicating the perfection or the completion of things and is used often as a symbolic way to describe wholeness.

The seven subtle bodies are well-known in Eastern religious philosophy, and their meaning and connotations have changed little over the centuries. Each of these bodies has its own function and purpose. It would be impossible in this practical book to cover all seven in detail, and there is no real need so to do, except to explain their important relationships and how their energy imbalances produce signs and symptoms within the physical body. Since the majority of people reading this book will have been indoctrinated into the Western system of medicine, I realize how difficult it will be for someone to have his or her mind changed (and hence his or her clinical practice) simply by reading something from a new perspective. This book explores a philosophy that is mostly alien to our Western-taught ideas of physiology, and what, over the centuries, has become second nature to Eastern mystics, yogis, and the like is almost impossible to rationalize or quantify using science. There seems to be an obsession today with scientifically proving anything and everything, merely because we live in a scientific age. Questions about scientific validation would not have arisen fifty years ago. Having said that, science *has* made enormous strides over the past few years in attempting to validate the "energy" body and energy medicine as a whole.

THE AURA

It is generally understood that there are seven subtle bodies, including the Physical, that make up the aura, or the energy field emanating from living beings. Some authorities place the seven subtle bodies outside the physical body. They are the Physical, Etheric, Emotional, Mental, Intuitional, Monadic, and the Divine. Different philosophies and individuals have given these bodies other names, depending on whether they are discussed in Eastern religious, Hindu, Buddhist, or Western spiritual terms. The seven names mentioned above are simply those generally adopted and accepted. There are also subdivisions of the etheric body, and there are said to be at least two more subtle bodies further out from the Spiritual, the gateways of which are bound by two more subtle body chakras. Some very gifted people (clairvoyants) are able to see and interpret auras. Some people can feel auras but not see them, and still others can see colors. In all my years of investigation and clinical practice, I have come to be able to see the etheric layer and can also "feel" most of them. It is important to get a grasp of these subtle bodies before being introduced to the chakras. Knowledge and acceptance of them are fundamental to being able to learn and use the chakras. One cannot exist without the other. Let's review them now.

The Physical Body

The physical body is the dense matter that is seen, touched, and felt by the majority of hands-on therapists. It is the one that we palpate, pummel, stroke, heat, or stick needles into. Looking at a person from a purely esoteric viewpoint, the physical or dense body has very little significance. A yogi or sage, for example, would not be interested in a physical body condition. To the rest of us mere mortals, however, it is the physical body that we treat using physical therapy, manipulation, acupressure, acupuncture, reflexology, biomagnetics, massage, craniosacral therapy, and so on. More important, it is the physical body that shows us the signs and symptoms of energy imbalance. Symptoms are golden pearls of information that are used by the practitioner in considering the *cause* of the disease and how steps can be taken to cure or balance the disease or condition.

Unless you are treating an obvious injury to the physical body, be it the result of a direct blow or repetitive strain, the *cause* of most disease is not within the physical body. Doctors can take blood samples, swabs, and cultures; surgeons can remove organs and perform intricate surgery in an attempt to heal, but they often perform these tasks in a misguided way. The physical body does *not* generally give the cause of disease (dis-ease)—it merely houses the symptoms. This point is extremely important and will be referred to again and again. Before you discard this book in sheer disbelief at the arrogance and treasonous statements I have made, let me assure you that treating the physical body with acupressure and other healing modalities through the chakras affects all the other subtle bodies and hence addresses the etiology, the true cause, of the disease or injury. What more could a healing practitioner want?

Of course, physical therapists treat and diagnose through the physical body and can achieve superb results by doing only this. Generally, though, many therapists treat mechanical conditions without necessarily thinking about whether the part of the body being treated has any connection to an endocrine gland, internal organ, or energy pathway, let alone a spiritual pathway. Each part of the physical body has all these associations, and when we become truly holistic practitioners, we should take all of them into account. It is not surprising, therefore, when the patient has certain reactions in areas of the body not being treated. The physical body has many areas of reflected pathways (that is, reflexes) that can be used in both diagnosis and treatment, some of which are already well-known in the traditional Oriental systems of medicine, applied kinesiology, and reflexology. When these reflected pathways are included in treatment, you will be able to make a truly holistic analysis and diagnosis, enabling you to assist the patient at a more in-depth level.

Physical therapists working with the physical body are all different and obviously take varied approaches. There are, sadly, a few bad practitioners, just as there are good and bad in every profession. These therapists are quite content to work at a purely local, symptomatic level. The experienced, conscientious physical therapist, however, will know, for instance, that a severe ankle inversion sprain that hasn't received any treatment will be followed in a short period of time by mechanical changes occurring elsewhere as a secondary effect. The muscles of eversion will become tight, causing possible subluxation of the talus and most certainly affecting the upper end of the fibula at the superior tibiofibular joint. In turn, this will create tension in the common peroneal nerve, the hip and sacroiliac joint, followed by pelvic tilting, thoracic scoliosis, and finally, atlas or even cranial misalignment.

Each of these mechanical deviations is the result of the original mechanical imbalance, and good osteopaths, chiropractors, or manipulative physical therapists can adjust the various joints in reverse order to produce alignment of the physical body. It is like peeling back the layers of the onion; the patient relives all the previous hurt, injury, and trauma that followed the original injury. This may occur in a transient way, with the patient almost unaware of changes, or the adjustments can have a huge impact.

The holistic therapist who appreciates that mind and body are *one*, and that the body is merely *energy* in various frequencies, will also know that in the same patient with an untreated ankle sprain, there will also be organic changes, initially with the bladder and the large intestine, possible skin irritation around the pudendum, then pain in the epigastric region, followed by a sore throat and finally dizziness, headache, or even tinnitus. The patient may also exhibit various emotional fluctuations between anxiety, fear, anger, and tearfulness. If you do not appreciate the emotional-physical tie-in, then you may think of patients who complain of such feelings and sensations following treatment as simply neurotic. You should also be aware that no symptoms be suppressed. Symptoms, which the patient exhibits to draw attention to the cause, are for guidance purposes only. They are not the disease itself, so they should never be suppressed with drugs, electrotherapy, symptomatic pain relief acupuncture, or any rub-on ointments unless you are treating a localized trauma.

The topic of mind-body relationships is a huge one and cannot be adequately covered in this book. It is, however, the subject of another book in the series, to be entitled *The Holistic Spine*, which will deal not only with the relationships between joints, muscles, organs, endocrine glands, and every vertebral level but also with how imbalances may be treated using physical therapy.

The Etheric Body
Structure

The word *etheric* comes from *ether,* meaning "the state between energy and matter." This is the first body that although it is called "invisible" can nonetheless be seen by clairvoyants and indeed most children up to the age of seven, who treat it as quite normal. All life forms possess an etheric body. Animals and plants especially are blessed with very rich etheric energy fields. Children have much more abundant natural energy at an etheric level than adults do, and it is for this reason that children and animals answer so much better to treatment using subtle energy approaches than adults.

Though the etheric body is invisible to most of us, with diligence, it is possible to "tune in" and see it. Following many intensive courses on the subject, even I have been able to detect the denser part of the etheric body. There are two parts to the etheric body, the *physical-etheric* and the *etheric-emotional.* The physical etheric consists of a network of fine tubular threadlike channels commonly known as the *nadis,* and these are related to the cerebrospinal fluid, endocrine glands, and the autonomic nervous system. The *nadis* will be covered in more detail later in the chapter. These two parts of the etheric body are in constant communion with each other and are usually thought of as just one subtle body.

The etheric body is a weblike structure that is in constant motion and to clairvoyants appears as a bluish-gray light moving at great speed and mingling with the other subtle bodies. Some of the more esoteric texts mention that the etheric body is an exact replica of the physical body, containing organs and tissues and so forth. The outer edge of the physical-etheric body is approximately three quarters of an inch (two centimeters) from the physical body, and the outer border of the etheric-emotional body is approximately four inches (eight to ten centimeters) from the physical body. These distances vary enormously with the age, gender, and well-being of the person. A very well-balanced individual has a different etheric makeup than someone who is ill. In areas of inflammation of the physical body the color of the etheric is usually rich in color, and where there is a chronic condition, the etheric energy is more translucent, also showing a congestion and dullness in color. Figure 1.1 shows the subtle bodies of the aura. This is also shown as Color Plate 1.

Functions

The etheric body has three main functions that are all closely related. It acts as receiver, assimilator, and transmitter of vital force via the chakras. In other words, it represents a vast clearinghouse of energy from inside out and from outside in; it also assimilates and sifts the energy. It is the largest "colander" that human beings possess. The individual chakras themselves, as will be discussed in detail in the next chapter, are energy gateways between the physical body and the subtle bodies.

Evidence

What evidence is there, apart from clairvoyant sight, proving the existence of the etheric body and the remainder of the aura (the subtler bodies)? In 1869 Dr. Walter Kilner, intrigued by the claims of clairvoyants, began researching the human electrical field by using dyes, a glass lens, and a screen and "proved" the aura could be seen. Though he detected only the first layer of the etheric body, it was a major triumph. The first person to succeed in taking photographs of the aura was the Croatian engineer Nikola Testa. His earliest photographs were of auras around the fingertips, but he later photographed the entire body. Tesla, who was also reputedly the founder of modern electrical power, used a large number of electrical wires attached to the body to make these images.

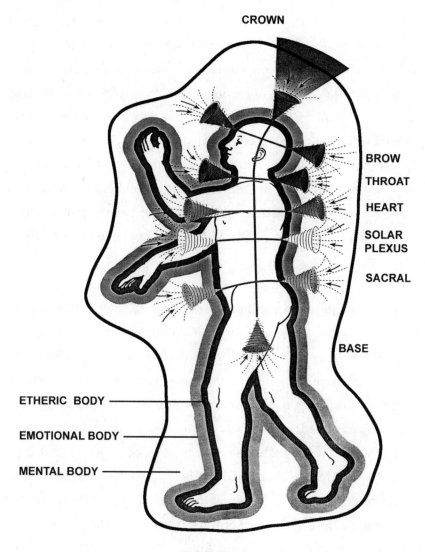

FIGURE 1.1
The Major Chakras and the Aura

In 1939 the Soviet scientists Semyon and Valentina Kirlian came up with a more practical way of photographing the aura by using electrical plates that emitted a current. The person placed his or her hand on the condenser plate, an electrical charge was transferred from the plate to the fingertip, and a photograph was taken. Kirlian photography is still used today. It has, however, largely been superceded by aura-imaging techniques developed by Guy Coggins and others in 1980. This technique makes use of a special camera to produce a full spectrum of colors of the aura. Aura-imaging cameras have become an increasingly popular way of discovering what the aura looks like at any given moment. One's aura changes according to mood, disposition, and physical illness, which means that to truly have a record of an individual's aura, several photographs have to be taken in a short space of time. Guy is now working on an aura-video system so that the subtle body may be seen in movement.

Feel

Since touch and feel are at the core of this book, before reading any further, it would be a good idea for you to practice "feeling" the etheric body. You may have done this already at weekend workshops. If not, here are some simple instructions. Sit in a comfortable, relaxed position. Try not to have any extraneous thoughts whirring round in your head, but keep a clear and focused mind. Place your palms together a few inches away from the body. Gently part them to about shoulder width, still opposed to each other. Now very slowly, bring the hands closer together until they are about one inch apart. Repeat the exercise two or three times. What did you feel? The majority of people will feel some kind of "barrier," albeit very subtle, when the hands are approximately four inches apart. Another barrier is often felt further out. Also, when the hands are brought very close together, a kind of buffer, similar to the poles of a magnet repelling each other, may be experienced. As a scientific test, this does not "prove" anything. It simply means that the majority of people who perform this exercise feel roughly the same thing. To me, though, this fact speaks volumes.

Paracelsus, sixteenth-century alchemist and physician, wrote of the etheric body: "Hence man has also an animal body and a sidereal [etheric] body, and both are one and not separated, the relationship between the two is as follows. The animal body, the body of flesh and blood, is in itself always dead. Only through the action of the sidereal body does the motion of life come into the other body. The sidereal body is fire and air, but it is also bound to the animal life in man, thus man consists of water, earth, fire and air."

David Tansley, in his groundbreaking book *Radionics and the Subtle Anatomy of Man*, describes the etheric body as consisting of "fine energy threads or lines of force and light and is the archetype upon which the physical body form is built. It can best be described as a field of energy that underlies every cell and every atom of the physical body by permeating and interpenetrating every part of it and extending beyond to form a part of what is called the health aura." The etheric body is simply the energy gateway to the physical body via the chakras producing an energy field within and without the physical. It has been called many things by different individuals and cultures throughout time. This force has been called *prana, chi, ki, medicatrix naturae, odic force, huna, animal magnetism, pneuma, archaeus, universal energy,* and *life force,* to mention just a few. In this book we will refer to it as vital force.

It is the manipulation of vital force within the etheric and physical bodies that brings about balance from imbalance, ease from disease, or harmony from disharmony. Within the etheric-fed physical body you can feel and use the vital force in many ways that will be discussed in this book. It can be with acupressure, reflexology, applied kinesiology, craniosacral therapy, various forms of soft tissue and joint mobilizing, and etheric healing. All these treatments are designed to bring about a balance of vital force within the individual.

Emotional (Astral) Body
Structure

The third body (and second subtle body) is generally called the emotional body because it involves our feelings. The border of its body is the same shape as that of the physical and etheric bodies, and it lies with an outer boundary of approximately ten to twelve inches (twenty to twenty-five centimeters) above the physical body. It does, however, intermingle with the etheric-emotional body and has an accentuated energy field around the top of the head and the mid-chest region. Its structure is much more fluid than that of the etheric, and most esoteric tomes agree that it does not duplicate the physical body. It appears to the clairvoyant as colored clouds of fine substance in continual fluid motion. The color is bluish-yellow near the rim of the etheric body, becoming more yellow-white toward the subtler region of the mental body.

Most clairvoyants (though not all in my experience) can see the emotional body, although it takes many days of painstaking focus and concentration for the those who are not naturally to perceive that there really is "something" more distant from the physical body than the etheric body. Barbara Ann Brennan, in her excellent book *Hands of Light*, writes,

This body interpenetrates the denser bodies that it surrounds. Its colors vary from brilliant clear hues to dark muddy ones, depending on the clarity or confusion of the feelings or energy that produces them. Clear and highly energized feelings such as love, excitement, joy, or anger are bright and clear; those feelings that are confused are dark and muddy. This body contains all the colors of the rainbow. Each chakra looks like a vortex of a different color and follows the colors of the rainbow.

These colors will be discussed further in Chapter 2.

Function

In the emotional body, multitudes of changes are constantly taking place, even if the individual is not appreciative of that fact. Each person is literally bombarded by stimuli of one sort or another from external and internal sources. The main function of the emotional body is to act as a filter, similarly to the etheric body, of stimuli coming toward the physical from the mental body and beyond and also of those stimuli created within the physical body. This process occurs without our knowledge; we are in blissful ignorance most of the time. It is only when an energy imbalance occurs in the emotional body or with the chakras that penetrate it that we are made aware that something is occurring.

The changes in our emotions can ultimately lead to changes, and hence symptoms, in the physical body. It is said that the vast majority of imbalance in the physical body are created by an aggravation of the emotional body. This aggravation, in turn, is caused by constant negative emotions, such as anger or fear, within the emotional body or the filtering of "thought forms" from the mental body. When a person has negative emotional feelings and sensations, even for a short while, the destructive potential created within the emotional body eventually affects that area of the physical body to which it is associated. Shyness and an inability to express one's emotions easily, for example, are quite often represented in disharmony of the Throat chakra, resulting in symptoms around the throat, shoulders, and large intestine. It is also said that the many viruses affecting the physical body via the chakras emanate from the emotional body. When there is strong and long lasting emotional imbalance, clairvoyants quite often see areas of dullness in the astral field that become more lucid and energetic with treatment. The emotional body is probably the most complex and the most active of all the subtle bodies.

Evidence

The emotional body is considered the highest of the "lower self" (a person's subtle body constitution), with the remaining four subtle bodies representing the "higher self" or our more "spiritual" aspect. Although proof of the existence of the emotional body has relied very heavily on the sightings of many hundreds of clairvoyants, the scientific evidence is scant. At one time it was thought that Kirlian photography was capturing the emotional body. Although this is now known not to be the case, claims have been made that aura-soma photography can depict the emotional body. Research in this area is ongoing.

Feel

It is relatively easy, with suitable training, to feel the emotional body. This is particularly true when feeling the boundaries between it and the etheric and the mental bodies. One can feel a definite sensation difference at the boundaries. The feeling on the therapist's hands are most acute when placed over the chakra at the emotional level (which is the size of a large plate at the emotional-mental border), but may also be felt at nonchakra parts of the body. These relative sensations will be discussed in the final chapter.

Mental Body
Structure

The mental body is said to be the lowest of the "higher," or spiritual, self. It can extend as much as thirty inches (seventy-five centimeters) from the physical body and is obviously much less dense than the bodies previously discussed. The fine substance that constitutes the mental body is whitish-yellow and has a very rapid vibrational rate compared with that of the denser bodies. It is this subtle body (and those beyond) that is used by spiritual healers in their "off-body" healing.

Function

The substance that makes up the mental body concerns thoughts and mental processes, sometimes called "thought forms." In simple language, when we think, this is the region where our thoughts originate. What we think affects us and those with whom we come into contact. If our natures are engendering, positive, and helpful, and we direct lots of lovely thoughts toward our fellow human beings (and ourselves), we feel well. In contrast, if we show negativity, hatred, pessimism, grief, sorrow, or depressive tendencies, these are eventually reflected in our physical makeup.

There is a hackneyed phrase that "we are what we eat," which to a certain extent is true, but it is even more true that *we become what we think.* Not only do we feel better within when we exhibit positive thought patterns but also, after a while the chemistry within the body changes; the blood chemistry, hormonal levels, and organic secretions all change. Many changes also take place within the autonomic nervous system, which then proceeds to affect the central nervous system. If we have nothing but negative thoughts, then we eventually destroy ourselves. *We are totally responsible for our own health,* or as much of our health as we have been granted at conception and birth, bearing in mind that various environmental factors may also affect us. This is a very simple philosophy—show compassion and love to all we meet, and be aware of shortcomings and failures. And try not to show egotism and selfishness, since these are both negative.

Evidence

As stated earlier, apart from the gifted clairvoyants, it is very difficult for most people to detect the mental body. Research is ongoing at the moment, and scientists are developing electrical apparatus capable of detecting the very high vibrations that exist within this body.

Feel

As with the emotional body, it is possible to feel the mental body. However, it takes a great deal of dedicated focus and training to do so. Like most things in life, practice makes perfect, and the more the potential therapist tries to feel the subtle bodies, the more he or she will succeed. The use of noncontact healing will be discussed in the final chapter.

The Intuitional, Monadic, and Divine Bodies

The three remaining subtle bodies are called the intuitional, monadic, and divine. These bodies are given several different names, depending on the philosophy and culture. Barbara Ann Brennan calls them the Etheric Template, the Celestial Template, and the Ketheric Template or the Causal body. The more esoteric or Buddhic literature calls them the Buddhic, Atmic, and Logoic, or Spiritual. It doesn't really matter what we call them. The important thing to realize is that each body is subtler and finer than its more proximal neighbor and that the chakras penetrate them all, thus providing a communion between a human being and his or her spiritual entity. It is beyond the scope of this text to describe these bodies further. If you wish to know more about them, many esoteric and metaphysical books that describe them more fully are available.

For those of you who have studied yoga, meditation, theosophy, anthroposophical medicine, or some of the Eastern religions, perhaps you are already familiar with much of what has been discussed so far. If, however, you have been wedded to a Western philosophy of medicine, you have had to take a deep breath to accept these theories at face value, just as I did many years ago. In time, you will come to acknowledge that the healing of our many ills comes from this knowledge. The many healing modalities, both subtle and physical, cannot be rationally explained without it.

THE CHAKRAS

The word *chakra* is Sanskrit for "wheel." The chakras are said to be "force centers" or whorls of energy permeating, from a point on the physical body, the layers of the subtle bodies in an ever-increasing fan-shaped formation. Rotating vortices of subtle matter, they are considered the focal points for the reception and transmission of energies. A clairvoyant can easily see these energy centers.

Each is different in form, makeup, color, and frequency. There are said to be seven major chakras, twenty-one minor chakras, and over seven hundred minichakras on the body that relate to acupuncture and major reflex points. The seven major chakras have contact with the physical body as single acupoints. Although most Eastern, Western, and New Age authorities accept that there are seven major chakras, it is apparent from research and personal experience that at least two other chakras exist that do not have direct contact with the physical body. They exist in the emotional body and beyond, above the Crown chakra. These will be discussed in the final chapter. Some authorities believe there are as many as nine major chakras and forty minor chakras, and others think there are as few as three majors and eight minors.

The study of chakras is lifelong. Indeed, the entire concept is based on many different philosophies and cultures, some of which will be considered in this book. Some authorities insist that the power to influence the chakras lies totally within the mind—as in kundalini yoga and some forms of meditation—while others dismiss this notion and say that energy can only be influenced through healing modalities. The main philosophies are Buddhic, Hindu, Theosophical, anthropomorphic, New Age, and various individual Western ideas based on a potpourri and combinations of these. This book deals with how the centers may be influenced with various disciplines of therapy, especially those based on the works of Alice A. Bailey (Theosophical) and David Tansley (Western), plus a few others. The majority of this book, however, is based on my own observations and experiences.

Structure

The structure of a chakra differs from chakra to chakra and depends on the age of the person in question. Its general shape can be likened to an inverted ice cream cone, with the narrow end "attached" to the physical body. The size of the chakra at the outer border of the etheric body is approximately two inches; at the outer border of the emotional body it is the size of a saucer, and at the outer border of the mental body it is the size of a small dinner plate. Therefore, it can easily be seen that at the subtler levels away from the body the various major chakras intermingle their energies. (Figure 1.1 and Color Plate 1 show the major chakras and their interpenetrating of the subtle bodies. See also Color Plates 2–8 showing a clairvoyant's interpretation of the chakras, as well as Figure 5.2.)

The Crown and Base chakras of a baby are shaped like those of an adult, whereas the remaining five chakras are small and round, since they do not fully function until a person reaches the age of seven or thereabouts. The Base or Root chakra is said to deal with conceptual or ancestral energy, and the Crown deals with our spiritual awareness. At the age of seven, the Sacral chakra begins to function properly. The Solar Plexus chakra and so on follow this. It is at this time that the shape of the chakra changes to the typical inverted ice-cream cone shape of the adult. In each chakra there are four or more components of rotating vortices that form smaller chakras, and they seem to be cylindrical in shape. It is these individual components that vibrate and resonate to a particular frequency. The lower chakras resonate somewhat slowly, while the Brow and Crown chakras resonate at a phenomenal rate. These differences can be felt with practice—indeed with enough practice you can feel the differences in different parts of the chakra at an etheric, emotional, or mental level and to ascertain what treatment is required. This will be discussed at greater length in Chapter 5.

The Base chakra consists of four rotating vortices, the Sacral Chakra has six, the Solar Plexus has ten, the Heart has twelve, the Throat has sixteen, the Brow has ninety-six, and the Crown has a staggering 972. This is why the Crown chakra is called the thousand-petaled lotus (except in actual fact it is twenty-eight short of the magic number). As well as being divided into four or more whirling spherical components, each chakra, it is said, has a central "core" with radiating segments, rather like the cornea and iris in the eye.

The most important aspect of the structure of each chakra for the therapist to know, whether treating in an on- or off-body mode, is that each chakra is very different in its anatomy and function. It is only by constantly feeling, sensing, and being aware of their differences in structure and functions that you will begin to grasp their clinical and therapeutic importance. The chakras really *do* exist. It is difficult in the extreme to extol the virtues of invisible subtle energy with very little scientific evidence. I strongly suggest that you attend a suitable workshop on the subject so that you can learn to *feel* them. It is impossible to practice just from reading a book. Having said that, if you follow the practical chapters diligently and start to use the chakras in harmonizing the physical body, you will not go wrong. Do not start by going straight to the emotional body—it will not work. We must learn to walk before we can run!

Functions

The chakras have three functions:

- to vitalize and harmonize the physical, etheric, and emotional bodies
- to facilitate the development of self-consciousness
- to transmit spiritual energy, thereby bringing the individual into a state of spiritual being

The first function is undertaken with the therapies taught in this book. This is true, to a certain extent, of the second function as well, in that with treatment, the patient is made more whole in mind, body, and spirit. The third function remains the purview of the meditation arts and the various forms of yoga.

According to Tansley, in *Radionics and the Subtle Anatomy of Man*, the chakras can become imbalanced in three different ways: by becoming congested, overstimulated, or uncoordinated. These states of imbalance often do not appear alone but in combination with another state. Let us explore these imbalances below.

Congestion

Congestion occurs when energy is not allowed to flow freely. This often happens when there is a sluggishness of vital force, or chi, in an area that in turn affects the lymphatic drainage, blood flow, nerve stimulation, and the flow of cerebrospinal fluid. This process can occur either from within to outward or outward to within. An example of the former would be eating too much saturated fat, which causes congestion in the stomach and small bowel, and eventually in the skin; this causes lymphatic congestion and endocrine imbalance, leading to congestion in the Solar Plexus chakra (as well as in the Throat chakra). An example of the latter state is when invading micro-organisms give rise to congestion of the Throat chakra, causing lymphatic congestion in the tonsils and possibly affecting the rest of the immune system. The feel of a congested chakra is different from the feel of the other two.

Overstimulation

A chakra can become overstimulated when too much energy is drawn into and through it. A fever is an expression of an overactive focal point of energy that is trying to disperse and flow outward into physical expression. An overabundant sex drive causes overstimulation of the Base and Sacral chakras. A person working constantly under fluorescent lighting will have an overstimulated Brow chakra, resulting in headaches and a general "muzzy" feeling.

Uncoordination

Uncoordination occurs between two associated chakras, creating a weakness in one of them, which eventually results in poor health. If the physical and etheric counterparts of the chakra are not well integrated, then debilitation and devitalization will take place. When a chakra becomes congested or overstimulated, it seeks support from its coupled chakra, which in turn can cause symptoms there. An example would be impotence caused by the uncoordination of the Throat and Sacral chakras.

Each major chakra is associated with an endocrine gland, an autonomic nerve plexus, an organ, and a meridian; there are scores of other couplings. The link between the "external" chakra and the internal organ is the *nadis*, the invisible web of energy that penetrates and permeates the physical frame. Richard Gerber, in his first book, *Vibrational Medicine,* wrote:

> The nadis are formed by fine threads of subtle energetic matter. They are different from the meridians, which actually have a physical counterpart in the meridian duct system. The nadis represent an extensive network of fluid like energies that parallel the body nerves in their abundance. In the Eastern yogic literature, the chakras have been metaphorically visualized as flowers. The nadis are symbolic of the petals and fine roots of the flowerlike chakras that distribute the life force and energy of each chakra into the physical body. Various sources have described up to 72,000 nadis or etheric channels of energy in the subtle anatomy of humans. These unique channels are interwoven with the physical nervous system. Because of this intricate interconnection with the nervous system, the nadis affect the nature and quality of nerve transmission within the extensive network of the brain, spinal cord and peripheral nerves. Dysfunction at the level of the chakras and nadis can, therefore, be associated with pathological changes in the nervous system.

Psychics describe the *nadis* as a web of tramlines of multicolored complexity. It would be wonderful to see the human body through the eyes of a psychic or a clairvoyant, who can truly tell what magnificent creations human beings are. All human beings, after all, are just *energy* in various forms and frequencies.

All Is Energy!

The phrase "all is energy" is often used, and how true it is. Everything on this planet above absolute zero emits a particular radiation that resonates at a certain frequency. Scientists have proved this beyond a doubt (see *Energy Medicine: The Scientific Basis* by James Oschman). Even the most dormant and seemingly dead material is alive in its molecular activity. So if we accept "all is energy" as a truism, then we can accept the futility of suppressing the symptoms of the physical body. Our deepest internal organs and bones are all energy and are all capable of growth, reproduction, and self-healing.

A practitioner can influence the healing process by using the chakras in every system of the body. As stated previously, most disease begins in the mental and emotional bodies; the effects of the "negative force" there are transmitted "downward" into the physical body via the chakras. There is no doubt that by using this knowledge and by using acupuncture, acupressure, reflextherapy, craniosacral therapy, massage, osteopathy, radiesthesia, homoeopathy, or even the "laying on of hands," practitioners can help the body heal itself at a much more accelerated rate than it would if other forms of treatment were being used. In this context the word *healing* simply means "to make whole." It does *not* mean "to cure." Whatever level of healing you choose, you are simply creating a balance out of an imbalance within the patient by using *their* energy systems. The therapist him- or herself never heals or cures anyone—and anybody who professes to do so is a charlatan.

LEVELS OF HEALING

The chakras may be used to heal at any level, ranging from the obvious mechanical imbalance to emotional and mental imbalance. Let's explore these levels of healing now.

The Physical Level

The treatment of physical symptoms is perfectly permissible if those symptoms originate from an injury or some kind of external force or blow. Repetitive stress syndromes are in this category; see my first book, *Acupressure: Clinical Applications in Musculo-Skeletal Conditions*, for full descriptions. Relieving pain that is caused by energy congestion, which we with our Western thinking would call vascular, lymphatic, or nerve congestion, with some kind of physical therapy, is acceptable. Many practitioners who have attended workshops in healing with the chakras still specialize only in the treatment of musculoskeletal conditions, and this is fine. Patients are treated at the level of the therapist's competence, and practitioners usually attract patients at the level they are meant to. This is not meant in any way to denigrate or patronize practitioners in this group. As will be made clear in later chapters, the healing of the physical body can be performed by using *only* chakra healing. You will be amazed!

The Etheric Level

Symptoms of the physical body that are caused by one or more states of imbalance of the chakras can be treated via the etheric body. The list of these symptoms is endless, and many conditions will be mentioned later in the book. A few that spring to mind at this point are osteoarthritis (not caused by a sequelae fracture around a joint), spinal displacements and peripheral joint misalignments, gastric and bowel disorders caused by poor eating habits, and so on. Treatment at this level can be performed through the use of gentle physical therapy, osteopathy, chiropractic, postural retraining, zero balancing, reflexology, craniosacral therapy, acupuncture, acupressure, shiatsu, herbs, and low-potency homeopathics. The gentler forms of these therapies are preferred, since the subtler the body to be balanced, the subtler the treatment that is needed.

This underscores the folly of using violent manipulative techniques with spinal and peripheral lesions; they really are not necessary. When we realize that everything is energy and that ultimately the body heals itself, the gentler and subtler the treatment regime we use the better the results will be. Also, the patient will not suffer from any of the post-treatment trauma or soreness that is normally endured with such treatment. Having said that, some patients actually like to receive heavy manipulative treatment, and they feel cheated if they have not been put into a "half nelson." Treatment at this level sometimes does meet a need.

The Emotional Level

As stated before, many disease patterns begin in the emotional body, so it is important for the therapist to be capable of dealing with the origins of disease. The conditions that fall into this category of healing are circulatory, neurological, gastric, renal, respiratory, and many muscular (yes, muscular!) ones. If this seems a little hard to swallow, just do a survey of all patients who complain of lumbar or upper-dorsal fibrositis with or without spinal lesions. You will find that these conditions are usually caused by stress or negative emotions. Therapies to tackle these conditions have to be geared to a subtler situation. These therapies would include acupuncture, acupressure, reflexology, metamorphic technique, craniosacral therapy, zero-balancing, biomagnetic therapy, color healing, sound therapy, yoga, meditation, healing, Reiki, radionics, and the middle to upper range of homeopathic remedies (30c to 1M).

As we know, just because the healing is channeled toward the emotional level does not mean that "hands-off" bodywork has to be performed. Of course, many therapists and healers do work at this level because they feel comfortable with it, and it works. It is not, however, mandatory to do so. The hands *can* be kept in contact with the physical body to affect the body at this level.

The Mental Level

Most of our psychosomatic and mental imbalance stems from the mental body. This imbalance might originate within the mental body itself or may be caused by an emotional body imbalance or by imbalance at a much finer and subtler level. Conditions such as depression, phobias and fears, insecurity, anxiety, and some allergies and paranoia may stem from the imbalance of energies at the mental level. The therapies that are best suited are healing (either noncontact or remote), metamorphic technique, hypnotherapy, meditation, Reiki, yoga, visualization, radiesthesia and radionics, psychotherapy, and very high homeopathic remedies (10M +). Therapies such as massage, acupressure, reflextherapy and acupuncture are still valid, however, for use in mental body imbalance, since the etheric and emotional pathways that link the mental body via the chakras may need to be cleared, balanced, and treated to enable this high order of healing to be more effective.

The chakras may be employed in any of a dozen of different therapies in order to treat and balance energy, thus treating the whole person. Ask any competent acupuncturist or homeopath, or indeed any good naturopath, which main guiding symptoms influence his or her decision to use a specific treatment or remedy. The homeopath will say that a strong guiding "mental" picture is all-important and that once the remedy is worked out (repetorized) and given to the patient, if it (the similimum) is correct, then in time *all* the patient's symptoms should disappear. The acupuncturist will consider the pulses, tongue, abdomen, and general demeanor of the patient before placing needles or administering moxa to the correct points to affect the flow of chi and thus balance the patient's energy system. The radionic practitioner will decide on the "rate" that will best balance that organ or area at which the treatment is aimed. The herbalist will choose the herb or herbs that best fits the totality of symptoms the patient is expressing. The osteopath, chiropractor, or physical therapist manipulates the soft tissue in a way that will best balance that part of the physical body to create harmony in the patient's mechanics, joints, muscles, and nerves.

TRUE HEALING

All these therapies are valid, and I have used all of them in healing. However, when we enter the world of healing through the chakras, only the radionic practitioner or "healer" would have had any previous experience or knowledge of this energy system. With this technique, since we are addressing the *cause* of the patient's disease or condition, we are involved in "true healing." Since most illness has its roots in the emotions, it is *only* by balancing and treating the chakras that we can isolate and treat the *cause* of the problem successfully.

The balancing and treatment of the individual chakras are based on several criteria of physical and emotional syndromes and, *each is as valid as the other*. This is because each symptom is a signal to you, the practitioner, that there is something wrong somewhere, and whatever level of healing you consider, with this type of approach all the other symptoms *will* be balanced and healed. This is a very bold statement to make and is not one that I make lightly, but after working with the chakra energy system for the past twenty-eight years, I can state it with the utmost conviction. It does not matter, therefore, if you are a practicing osteopath and wish to continue using osteopathy or change to another modality. It does not matter if you are a practicing reflexologist and wish to continue using reflexology or change to another mode. Every type of hands-on therapy is catered to within the chakra energy system, and each is as valid and as important as each other. This cannot be overstated!

Therefore, regardless of your practice, you can use one or more of the following criteria to help formulate a treatment regimen. Look for the presence of the following:

1. An obvious imbalance of the physical parts of the body associated with and governed by a particular chakra. An example of this would be a lung condition treated via the Throat chakra.

2. An obvious imbalance with an endocrine gland associated with a particular chakra. An example of this would be estrogen imbalance treated by the Sacral chakra.

3. An obvious skeletal imbalance associated with a particular chakra. An example of this would be a mid-dorsal lesion treated with the Heart chakra.

4. An obvious muscular imbalance associated with a particular chakra. An example of this would be psoas major imbalance treated with the Base chakra.

5. An obvious or subtle emotional state associated with a particular chakra. An example of this would be anger or rage treated with the Brow chakra.

6. An imbalance of chi energy, felt through pulse diagnosis, in a particular meridian associated with a chakra. An example of this would be spleen meridian imbalance treated with the Sacral chakra. (For those of you who do not use or have never heard of pulse diagnosis, do not despair; there are other simple ways of testing meridian chi flow and chakra energy flow, to be covered in a later chapter).

7. A subtler (almost sixth-sense) perception that a chakra is in a state of imbalance and needs to be balanced and treated. Some very gifted people can *see* the states of the aura and the energy centers and *know* what treatment is needed. They can see the various energy vibrations, colors, and different densities of the subtle bodies. Others who cannot easily see these things become more adept over the years at actually *feeling* the energy patterns. The sensation of *touch* is used in the analysis, diagnosis, and subsequent treatment. Although it is useful to have this intuition, beware that students or therapists who are just learning these methods will ask you the reasons for using a particular technique and will not be satisfied when you tell them, "We just do it—but we do not know why."

In all these diagnostic and treatment rationales, each of the traditional methods of diagnosis can be used, as well as the more conventional ones. It is rare for just one chakra to be in a state of imbalance at any one time. Usually three and quite often more major and minor chakras (centers) need to be balanced and treated. It goes without saying that the more balancing and treatment that needs to be done, the more chronically sick the patient. Although it does not matter which type of diagnosis is used, there is obviously an order to the importance of symptoms:

1 mental, emotional, or psychosomatic symptoms

2. chi energy imbalance (diagnosed via the reflected pathways)

3. endocrine imbalance

4. physical or organic symptoms

5. skeletal imbalance

6. muscular symptoms

I have purposely omitted "sixth sense" from this list, since it does not fall within the scope of the book.

The words *open* and *closed* are often used in conjunction with the condition of a chakra. This is a simplistic, and often misleading, view of the energetic state of the chakras. If something is *closed*, it should mean that it is not functioning at all, whereas what is really meant is that a chakra in a state of sluggishness or congestion that needs to be stimulated. The word *open* is used to refer to a state of normality and harmony. These terms are used by psychics and those who meditate and do not have any useful clinical meaning. Although it is possible to affect the energetic condition of each chakra purely with the mind and intention, it is palpably impossible to *open* and *close* them at will.

THE ETIOLOGY OF DISEASE

Before you begin with analysis and treatment, it is very important that you understand in the broadest terms the cause of disease, as well as the principles involved and the rationale behind them. The causes of disease were discussed fully in my last book *Acupressure and Reflextherapy in the Treatment of Medical Conditions*. Below I will cover the most salient points.

It has now been firmly established that many the illnesses suffered by human beings have their roots in the mental or emotional bodies and that the disease pattern is filtered down through the etheric body and into the physical body via the chakras to present as physical symptoms. There are two general ways that disease can occur, internally and externally; the rest are variations of these two.

Internal Disease

Internal disease is either congenital, hereditary, or a reaction to certain stimuli.

The founder of modern homeopathy, Samuel Hahnemann, classified the causes of all chronic disease as three inherited taints, or "miasms," those of Psora, Syphilitic, and Psychotic. My classical homeopathic training has proved on countless occasions that Hahnemann's hypothesis is correct. In Hahnemann's time (the nineteenth century) there was no knowledge of genes and genetic coding. It is now known, however, that each person is born with a particular genetic blueprint that determines his or her weaknesses or strengths. It is possible, therefore, for a person born with a weakness that gives rise to the symptoms of, say, eczema, which appears because of some kind of shock or injury to the system, either through accident, injury, poison (as in food), grief, and so on. The actual eczema is dormant at birth; the person is born with the taint or predisposition, which then materializes in symptoms after the "jarring" has taken place. Hahnemann put it beautifully when he said that the "miasm is raised."

In the case of eczema, the taint or miasm of Psora is active; in the case of ulceration, the miasm of Psychosis is active; and in the case of glandular fever the Tubercular miasm (a combination of Psora and Syphilis) is active. The miasms represent a long and complicated study to which Hahnemann dedicated several years of his life. It is said that the Base chakra can influence the miasms. Indeed, it is the Base chakra that represents the conceptual and ancestral energy, which is the energy quality and quantity given to us before birth. You would do well to purchase a book on homeopathic philosophy—you will not regret it.

Many acute and febrile symptoms are caused by our body's reaction to certain poisons. Symptoms such as catarrh, irritable bowel syndrome, mouth sores, skin rashes, tonsillitis, behavioral imbalances, sweating, and tiredness can all be caused by adverse reactions to food. The body uses the immune system, the skin, and the bowel to rid itself of poisons. If this can be diagnosed, then the patient should omit the food or foods causing the sensitivity or allergy should be omitted from the diet for a period of at least three months, and you should treat him or her via the Throat or Solar Plexus chakra.

Another form of imbalance that causes internal symptoms is represented by many of the psychosomatic disorders. Many symptoms occurring in adulthood stem from how we were treated as children or adolescents; many energy imbalances are caused by our reaction then, or later, to the stresses and strains of that time in our lives. Through careful questioning and counseling you should be able to ascertain the root causes. These are mostly treated by a combination of the Brow and Heart chakra and to a lesser degree of the Solar Plexus chakra. The symptoms of this form of imbalance do not always show up as psychosomatic ones. They can sometimes be seen as physical symptoms, such as a "frozen" shoulder, lower back pain, or stomach cramps, to give just three examples. Careful questioning is important in ascertaining if there has been an accident or injury that might have caused the physical symptoms. If the answer to that question is in the negative, then you should start to look for another cause. I have encountered many cases of "frozen" shoulder that have been caused by a faulty diet or by some psychological problem such as introversion or shyness.

These examples may seem a little bizarre at first, but there are valid explanations for each. In the case of faulty diet, in which the person has a high intake of carbohydrates and fats, the toxins that the body is attempting to get rid of accumulate in the organs and excretion meridians. Thus the lungs and small and large intestines, as well as the lymphatic channels and drainage areas, become congested. All these channels are situated around the shoulder. The expression "not being able to shoulder responsibility" is one of several that have been passed down through the ages that point to symptoms derived from emotional causes. Asking the right questions during the initial consultation with a patient is all-important. Some training in psychology can help you to lead the questioning in the right direction.

External Disease

External forces cause external disease. Skeletal, muscular, and joint injuries, along with local wounds caused by external trauma, are the only types of imbalance that can be treated locally without causing imbalance in other systems of the body. Sprains and strains can be treated very effectively with localized physical therapy, although it is advisable to treat as early as possible so as to ascertain the extent of the injury and also to check the "whole" person after treatment when the obvious symptoms have been addressed. Some physical therapists and osteopaths are guilty of treating just the body part without considering everything else. Once treatment is finished it is essential that you "balance up" the injured part to the rest of the body. There are some simple and effective ways to do this, some of which will be discussed later in this book. Remember the example of the badly treated sprained ankle discussed earlier in the chapter that could have so many ramifications.

Often in life we undergo physical or emotional traumas. Unless we react to the trauma soon after the event, the shock and reaction stays within the system to become a "block" or a watershed. The latest medical research accepts that each cell has a memory. Traumas and accidents are memorized and stored by the body. Patients are often heard saying that they have never been well since the whiplash injury, the death of a parent, the steroids they took, the vaccination, and so on. Each of these represents a "block" to treatment and should be dealt with before the main part of the treatment commences.

When the block is a physical injury, the patient will "unwind" the injury with treatment. If an external agent such as shock or a virus has caused the block, a "letting go" will occur with the treatment. Some viral infections represent major stumbling blocks and can wreak havoc in the system if not dealt with quickly. Viruses can cause utter devastation within the human body. It never ceases to amaze me how something so small can reap so much havoc. The simple reason is that most viruses are foreign to the human energy system. According to Dr. Sir Fred Hoyle, who wrote *Diseases from Space*, viruses are not of this world. He maintains that most of them enter the earth's atmosphere via meteors and ice particles. In his book Hoyle outlines the incidences of influenza and other contagious diseases along certain geographical lines over which comets flew, spreading their debris. It is because viruses are alien to the human body that they are so difficult to treat correctly.

VITAL FORCE

The analysis of every type of etiology may be viewed as changes that take place in the person's vital force, or chi energy.

Vital force, or life force, is the energy makeup of the body. It permeates and interpenetrates every cell in the body and every part of the aura. Without it, we would not exist. We would not live or breathe. In my first two books I made much of one of the terms used to describe vital force, namely, *chi*. This was because these books predominantly covered the hands-on healing method of acupressure, a healing technique of Traditional Chinese Medicine (TCM). What is the relationship between the chi energy that flows within the meridians of the physical body and the energy of the chakra system? The straight answer is that no one knows. Therapists and healers have taken for granted that when the chakras are treated, the organs and meridians will be affected.

What about the other forms of life force that are said to have influence on the body, such as biophotonic energy, bioelectrical energy, and simple metabolic energy; how do they all fit in? Some therapists would insist that they are all the same, while others would state that a huge incompatibility exists between the different energy types. The simplistic answer, when we accept that "all is energy" is that by using the chakras, we *know* for certain that they are influencing *all* the other energetic systems of the body. In his excellent book *Vibrational Medicine for the 21st Century*, Richard Gerber discusses these different types of bioenergy in what he calls the "multidimensional human being." He enumerates four types of bioenergy: metabolic, bioelectrical, biophotonic, and subtle bioenergies (subtle magnetic life energies).

1. Metabolic energy has its source in food (fats, sugars, proteins),

which is converted by the body into ATP-cellular-energy currency. It is located throughout the cells of the physical body and is used to power basic cellular processes.

2. Bioelectrical energy has its complex source in the nerves, muscles, heart, GI tract, brain, bone matrix, and cellular mitrochondria. It is transmitted through the cells of the nervous system, muscles, organs, weight-bearing bones, and intercellular matrix. Bioelectrical energy is used in the movement of blood, food, and urine; in communication between the organs and nervous system; in assisting bone strength; and in local repair of tissue damage following infection or trauma.

3. Biophotonic energy has its source in UV biophotons emitted by DNA in the cell nucleus. It is located within the nuclei of all cells of the body and is used in cell-to-cell communication.

4. Subtle bioenergies (subtle magnetic life energies) constitutes the most complicated of the groups, in that it is the least well documented. Gerber subdivides this form of energy into *prana,* etheric energy, emotional energy, mental energy, and higher spiritual energy.

Prana is an environmental nutritive subtle energy that is carried by oxygen and sunlight and that flows through the chakras and *nadis* to provide energetic support for the organs and body tissues. Etheric energy, which he states is equivalent to basic life energy, or vital force, flows through the chakras of the etheric body and provides subtle energetic growth template for the physical body. Emotional energy flows through the emotional body and its chakras as emotional "thought forms." Mental energy flows through the mental body and its chakras as mental "thought forms" and is involved in intellectual functioning, creativity, and abstract thought. Higher spiritual energy flows through the higher spiritual bodies of "light" and is used as the flow of "soul" energy into physical form.

Dr. Gerber's classifications of energy show a well-researched and scientifically rational explanation of the various forms of energy that exist within and without the human body. Research into the many and varied frequencies that exist on areas of the body and that seem to exert a different electromagnetic influence—namely, the acupoints and major reflex points—is also being done.

What, in scientific terms, makes an acupoint both clinically useful and powerful, and what causes it to have no clinical value whatsoever? Following in that vein, why are the major and minor chakras positioned where they are? After all, on the physical body they are represented as acupoints no larger than the head of a pin. Before answering this question, it must be stated that the positioning of the major chakras is traditionally regarded as correct in most philosophies. Having said that, the exact acupoint placing is my own work—derived from a mixture of clinical research, common sense, and intuition. The positioning of the minor chakras was much more arduous—this process will be explained in the next chapter.

The power and efficacy of the acupoints lie in work that has been done in the field of bioenergetic profiling of the human body, with particular reference to energy frequencies. It is known that healing occurs at different frequencies. For example, nerve regeneration occurs at 2 hertz, bone growth at 7 hertz, ligament healing at 10 hertz, and so on. It is also known that some people are hypersensitive to certain frequencies, that is, the smell or ingestion of some chemicals can cause some people to feel very ill. This means that both disharmony and harmony exist at the many different frequencies. It is also known that the earth's magnetic frequency ranges between 7 and 10 hertz, with a mean average 7.8 (known as the Schumann resonance).

This frequency is also that of the Alpha-Theta state (A/T state), which occurs when there is harmony and healing between healer and patient. Research has shown that the frequency of connective tissue is the same as that of the brain. This is a wonderful scientific reinforcement of the beliefs that have been held for some time by contact therapists. It is now a known fact that when connective tissue is influenced either by subtle or stimulating means, this affects the brain and the central nervous system. Indeed, it is the autonomic nervous system that is first affected by therapies such as massage and aromatherapy. What is even more remarkable is that the A/T state of healing, harmony, and oneness is at the same frequency as the physical counterpart of the anterior Heart chakra. This point is at Conception 17 (Con 17) in the middle of the sternum. As will be discussed later, the Heart chakra is used in healing emotional and mental imbalance. If the therapist can produce the A/T state at the Heart chakra by resonating it and the patient's nervous system at approximately 7.8 hertz, then calmness, harmony, relaxation, and emotional healing should take place. Dr. Cyril Smith has made an in-depth study of the frequencies of acupoints. Table 1.1 on page 40 shows the chakra frequencies as found by Dr. Smith.

From the table, we can see that there is an approximate decrease in frequency rates, in ascending order. The exception to this is the Throat chakra, which has the same frequency as the Base and Sacral chakras (to be explained in the next chapter). It is not necessary to remember the individual frequencies, except that of the Heart chakra. It is interesting to note that the Heart is at the very center of a person.

TABLE 1.1. CHAKRA FREQUENCIES

Chakra	Minimum Frequency Range	Maximum Frequency Range
Crown	0.245	0.265
Brow	2.88	3.04
Throat	79.9	82.4
Heart	7.68	7.92
Solar Plexus	21.8	24.4
Sacral	79.9	82.4
Base	79.9	82.4

This is true for the spinal equivalent as well—the posterior Heart Chakra has its physical link with T6-T7, which is the very center of the spine.

It has already been mentioned that the understanding of the chakra energy system is based on several different philosophies. The quote below, based on Buddhic philosophy, represents a truly esoteric viewpoint. In it Michio Kushi explains the phenomenon of Heaven's Force entering the body via the Crown chakra and Earth's Force dispersing and entering via the Base chakra and the feet:

In the case of the human body, Heaven's Force enters the head (Crown) producing the aura. After entering the head, Heaven's Force intensively charges the inner regions of the brain, sending electromagnetic influences to millions of cells. Because of these charges distributed to all parts of the brain, these cells, organized in each region of the brain operate as highly communicative instruments and receive various sorts of vibration as well as electro-magnetic impulses producing images. Heaven's Force continuously descends forming the uvula at the deep inner region of the mouth cavity. The Force is then transmitted to the root of the tongue and the throat region, including the vocal chords. It further descends to the heart where the external muscles of the heart are activated and the charge there distributed to the circulatory system of the blood and lymphatic system in the same way that charges are distributed from the mid brain to all brain cells. Heaven's Force then descends to the stomach region to distribute to the surrounding organs such as the pancreas and spleen, the liver gallbladder and the kidneys.

Accordingly these organs produce various liquids, which are charged electromagnetically, including gastric acid, pancreatic juice, bile as well as local hormones. Heaven's Force continues to descend and intensively charges the lower part of the small intestine. Because of this charge, distributed throughout the small and large intestine in the form of waves, these organs move by contracting and expanding. Intestinal digestion, decomposition and absorption of food molecules as well as movement of food and bowels become possible because of these distributed forces. The Force further descends charging the lower part of the body including the bladder and the genitals. The function of the bladder, collecting and eliminating urine, and the functions of the genital area, producing and eliminating reproductive cells, results from the charge of these electro-magnetic forces. Heaven's Force then produces another "uvula" in the form of the penis or clitoris.

On the other hand, the Force from the Earth ascends from the ground towards Heaven, passing through the same channels through which Heaven's Force descends. Earth's Force enters the body through both feet. It also enters the lower parts of the body including the genital area, creating a unique form of indentation, the prostate gland in man and the uterus and ovaries in woman. Earth's Force continues to ascend and intensify its charge colliding at the abdominal wall and area with Heaven's Force. This accelerates various intestinal activities, including the secretion of intestinal juice and the gonad hormones. The Earth's Force continues to ascend and generates energies to the stomach, pancreas, spleen, liver and gallbladder. Ascending further, the heart region is charged and cardiac movement is made possible by the combination of the two forces. The Force of the Earth vibrates the vocal chords then, reinforcing the breathing function and accelerating tongue activity as well as releasing charges into the mouth cavity (unity of the Conception and Governor meridians). Because of this, high-pitched sound can be created and inhalation can be made and faster motion of the tongue is facilitated. Earth's Force is then transmitted towards the brain region, and charges its center, the mid brain and millions of brain cells. The Heaven's Force tends to charge the right side of the brain, whilst the earth's Force the left side. The parts of the body where the forces collide and form union are called the *chakras*. These places are each generating electro-magnetic flow towards the outside and at the same time are receiving invisible force from the surrounding atmosphere to charge the internal functions.

What a marvelously descriptive piece of writing that is. It offers some theories about the formation of the chakras on the physical-etheric level as well as much esoteric physiology that we, as therapists, should do a little more than just ponder.

CHAPTER TWO

The Chakras

Now that we have explored the subtle anatomy of the aura and chakras in general, let's turn to an in-depth examination of the chakras.

THE SEVEN MAJOR CHAKRAS

In his book *The Chakras*, first published in 1927, the Theosophist the Reverend C. W. Leadbetter placed the major chakras on the front of the body. Tibetan and Sanskrit literature, on the other hand, places them on the spine. Djwal Khul, a fourteenth-century philosopher, says that they lie some three inches behind the spinal column. David Tansley states that they are found on the anterior aspect, whereas Barbara Ann Brennan, in her book *Hands of Light*, places them front and back. St. John the Divine, in his Book of Revelation, writes of seven seals on the back of the book of life, referring to the force centers and their placement. The truth is, *it does not really matter*, since each placement is correct, according to the individual's philosophy and practice. My experience is similar to Brennan's; each chakra has a dorsal and ventral aspect, and the influence of the chakra *girdles* the body at that given level. It is, however, at the spinal and frontal aspects where there is more focus of energy, and this is why these aspects are usually chosen in treatment. Of the two, the spinal aspect deals mostly with musculoskeletal and "yang" imbalance, whereas the ventral aspect deals mostly with organic, emotional and "yin" imbalance.

The chakras, with their relative spinal positions and ventral acupoint locations are as follows:

TABLE 2.1. THE POSITIONING OF THE SEVEN MAJOR CHAKRAS

Chakra	Spinal Level	Spinal Acupoint	Ventral Acupoint
Crown		Gov 20	Gov 20
Brow	Occipito-Atlas	Gov 16	Extra 1 (Yintang)
Throat	C7-T1	Gov 14	Con 22
Heart	T6-T7	Gov 10	Con 17
Solar Plexus	T12-L1	Gov 6	Con 14
Sacral	L4-L5	Gov 3	Con 6
Base	Sacrococcyx	Gov 2	Con 2

I have abbreviated the Governor and Conception vessels as Gov and Con respectively to avoid the confusion that sometimes occurs with the use of GV and CV or of the variations of Du Mai and Ren Mai, as used in TCM. Modern acupuncture meridian abbreviation nomenclature is used for the other meridians.

Although, strictly speaking, the chakra is situated in the auric field above the physical body, a focal point of energy is at the center of the chakra that is positioned on the skin at an acupoint. It is therefore possible, as mentioned earlier, to affect the energies both at a physical level and an etheric level at the same time by using the therapies discussed in this book.

Associations and Correspondences

Each of the seven major chakras (sometimes called "centers") is associated with up to twenty-two different correspondences. Although it is not important to know them all, a complete study of them is fascinating. At each chakra there is an anatomical position (ventral); anatomical position (dorsal); acupoints dorsal and ventral; Sanskrit terminology and interpretation; symbol; coupled major chakra; coupled minor chakra; endocrine gland association; organic association; spinal-level association; "key" points; associated meridians; associated spiritual phenomena; muscular association; autonomic nerve association; color and sound correspondences; and a differing number of rotating vortices. There are also many other associations and relationships, which are outside the scope of this book. These include Element, Life Lesson, Gemstone, Essential Oil, Crystals, Herbs, Earth Energy, Planet, and Metal.

Anatomical Positions

The anatomical positions are given in both acupoint and anatomical terms and represent the point on the physical body (skin) that is usually the center of the influence of the chakra. Although an exact point is given for each chakra, it differs sometimes with certain individuals, just as acupoints can vary. There is an area of influence around each major and minor chakra point just as there is around ordinary acupoints. This is important to realize when the whole hand is placed over the chakra (as sometimes occurs clinically), but usually just a finger pad is used. Experience tells you that there is much more effect when you are "spot-on" the point. (See Figure 2.1.)

Sanskrit

Sanskrit, an ancient Indo-Aryan language and the classical language of India and of Hinduism, is still used today. Each major chakra has a corresponding Sanskrit term:

- Crown: The Sanskrit is *Sahasrara* and means "thousand-petaled" and also "dwelling place without support."
- Brow: The Sanskrit is *Ajna* and means "authority, command, and unlimited power."
- Throat: The Sanskrit is *Vishuddha* and means "pure."
- Heart: The Sanskrit is *Anahata* and means "unstricken."
- Solar Plexus: The Sanskrit is *Manipura* and means "the city of gems."
- Sacral: The Sanskrit is *Svadhisthana* and means "dwelling place of the self."
- Base: The Sanskrit is *Muladhara* and means "foundation."

Symbol

The symbols used for each chakra are Hindu in origin and are mostly used as focal objects for meditation. In descending order from Crown to Base, they are Lotus, Star, Crescent, Cross, Circle, Triangle, and Square. Some more elaborate symbols, which relate to animals such as the elephant and crocodile, are also used in both Hindu and Buddhic cultures. The shape and form of these symbols depend on country, culture, history—and personal preference. These symbols, however, are generally esoteric and should not concern the hands-on practitioner.

Coupled Major Chakra

The relationships between major chakras are often used in clinical practice to balance the energies in each center:

- The Crown chakra is associated with the Base chakra.
- The Brow chakra is also associated with Base chakra.
- The Throat chakra is associated with the Sacral chakra.
- The Heart chakra is associated with the Solar Plexus chakra.

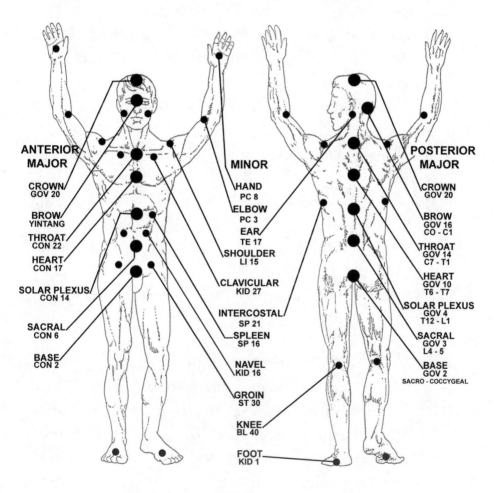

FIGURE 2.1

Anatomical Positions of the Major and Minor Chakras

Please note that the Base is associated with the top two chakras, the Crown and the Brow. Full details on practical applications will be provided later.

Coupled Minor Chakra

Each major center is associated with a minor center, the latter being the center's reflected point of energy as well as a powerful acupoint in its own right:

- The Crown chakra is associated with the Foot and Hand chakras.
- The Brow chakra is associated with the Clavicular and Groin chakras.
- The Throat chakra is associated with the Shoulder and Navel chakras.
- The Heart chakra is associated with the Ear and Intercostal chakras.
- The Solar Plexus chakra is associated with the Spleen chakra.
- The Sacral chakra is also associated with the Spleen chakra.
- The Base chakra is associated with the Knee and Elbow chakras.

These relationships are used a great deal in clinical practice and will be dealt with more fully later.

Endocrine Gland

Each of the seven major chakras is related to an endocrine gland. This is possibly the most important relationship to learn and understand. Its significance in clinical work is enormous, as are the theoretical and practical ramifications. Although in the esoteric literature, this relationship is scantily dealt with, it is one of the most concrete associations that can be reproduced and used in therapy again and again to produce spectacular clinical results. The endocrine glands are obviously part of the physical body and have nerve, blood, lymphatic, and energy links to the physical body and yet produce natural chemicals (hormones) that can be extremely powerful in affecting the physical, etheric, and emotional bodies. The esoteric literature states that the *nadis* is the mediation between the etheric chakra and the physical endocrine gland (see Chapter 1). The advent of craniosacral therapy and other hands-on subtle therapies has proved this link beyond a doubt. The relationships between chakras and endocrine glands are as follows:

- The Crown chakra is associated with the pineal gland.
- The Brow chakra is associated with the pituitary gland.
- The Throat chakra is associated with the thyroid and parathyroid glands.
- The Heart chakra is associated with the thymus gland.
- The Solar Plexus chakra is associated with the pancreas gland.
- The Sacral chakra is associated with the ovaries and testes.
- The Base chakra is associated with the adrenal medulla and the adrenal cortex.

Please note that the Brow chakra is also associated with the thalamus and hypothalamus areas of the brain. The relationship between the Base and Sacral chakras and their corresponding endocrine glands as presented here represent my own findings and are somewhat contrary to what is mentioned in other publications. These findings will be explained later in the chapter when the individual chakras are discussed. (See Figure 2.2.)

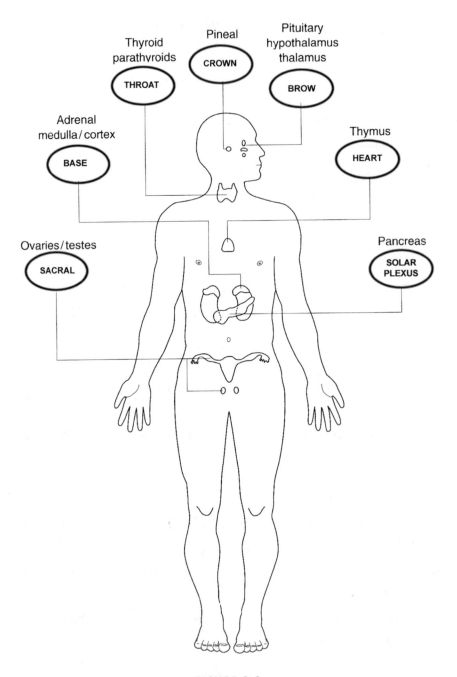

FIGURE 2.2

Associations of the Major Chakras with the Endocrine Glands

Associated Organs

Each major chakra is related to one or more internal organs or parts of the body. This knowledge is vital in clinical terms. The chakras relate to the organs/body parts via the meridian energy system, either through the main twelve bilateral meridians or the eight extraordinary ones:

- The Crown chakra is associated with the upper brain (higher functions) and the right eye.
- The Brow chakra is associated with the lower brain (brain and nervous system), ears, nose, and the left eye.
- The Throat chakra is associated with the lungs, bronchus, throat, larynx, pharynx, upper lymphatics, and large intestine.
- The Heart chakra is associated with the heart, blood circulation, middle lymphatics, and the vagus nerve.
- The Solar Plexus chakra is associated with the stomach, liver, spleen, pancreas, gallbladder, and duodenal/jejunum parts of the small intestine.
- The Sacral chakra is associated with the reproductive system, lower lymphatics, and ileum part of the small intestine.
- The Base chakra is associated with the spinal column, kidneys, and bladder.

Associated Meridians

Each major chakra is related to one, two, or three meridians, and each minor chakra is related to just one. These relationships may be used in several ways. They can be used as a "backup" energy system in balancing and treatment. They can be used at the start of a treatment in sedating or stimulating the related organ or body part. Once again, these relationships are my interpretation based on several years of practical experience. The eight extraordinary meridians are included in parentheses. These are used when giving acupuncture with the chakras. They relationships between the chakras and the meridians are as follows:

- The Crown chakra is associated with the Triple Energizer meridian.
- The Brow chakra is associated with the Gallbladder meridian (Yangwei Mai).
- The Throat chakra is associated with the Large Intestine and Lung meridians (Yangchiao Mai).
- The Heart chakra is associated with the Heart and Small Intestine meridians (Yin Wei Mai).
- The Solar Plexus chakra is associated with the Liver and Stomach meridians (Dai Mai).
- The Sacral chakra is associated with the Spleen and Pericardium meridians (Yinchiao Mai).
- The Base chakra is associated with the Bladder and Kidney meridians (Conception, Governor and Chong Mai).

Key Points

When using the chakra energy system with acupuncture, the Key points, those related to each chakra (two for a major chakra and one for a minor), are needled first in order to "open up" the energy center. They are used in a similar way to the Key points of the eight extraordinary meridians. The Key points lie both on the midline and on the body periphery. When used with acupressure and reflextherapy, they balance and treat the chakra and are a part of the whole treatment. In touch therapy, only the peripheral associated Key points need be used. In the following list the other Key points used in acupuncture are shown in parentheses:

- The Crown chakra Key point is TE 5 (Con 4).
- The Brow chakra Key point is SP 6 (Gov 4).
- The Throat chakra Key point is LR 5 (Con 6).
- The Heart chakra Key point is HT 1 (Gov 7).
- The Solar Plexus chakra Key point is TE 4 (Con 17).
- The Sacral chakra Key point is PC 3 (Gov 12).
- The Base chakra Key point is LR 8 (Con 22).

These chakra Key points are based on my own research. When I was doing my acupuncture doctoral thesis in 1987, I maintained that these points were useful only in acupuncture. Further research, though, has revealed that they are of significant practical importance in acupressure as well. I originally found these points through a combination of trial and error, dowsing, and common sense. Looking back, I can't imagine what some of my poor patients went through as I attempted to verify the accuracy of these points! The use of acupuncture and the chakra system of energy will be fully covered in the next book in the series.

Associated Muscles

The treatment of musculoskeletal lesions is just one aspect of this amazing therapy. The advent of applied kinesiology (AK) has heightened our awareness of the integration between meridian energy flow and muscular innervation, as well as organic-muscular associations. My own research has taken this one stage further by relating various muscles to each of the major chakras. In practical terms, muscles may now be strengthened, weakened, or simply treated in a very rapid and easy way by balancing the muscle with the chakra. Details of how to balance muscle energy using applied kinesiology appear in the book on acupressure in the treatment of musculoskeletal conditions. A full table of muscle-major chakra-minor chakra relationships will appear in Chapter 3.

Associated Reflexes

As with any part of the body, the physical aspects of the chakras have reflected points or reflexes. In practical terms, the important ones appear on the feet and hands, but they also appear on the arms and legs. This approach, of using the reflected chakras on the feet, called "light touch reflexology (LTR)," is my own invention and is described in Chapter 4.

Associated Emotions

Each major chakra is also associated with an emotion or emotions. Each emotion may be used as part of the diagnostic armamentaria in recognizing which chakra may be in a state of imbalance. Conversely, the chakra healing techniques may be used to highlight the emotional cause of an illness. As stated previously, a high percentage of conditions, diseases, and illnesses have emotional causes. When receiving treatment that combines the chakras with acupressure, reflexology, and/or craniosacral therapy, the patient often experiences an emotional release that may or may not be directly linked with the chakra being treated. The release may be manifest as anger, tearfulness, sighing, yawning, even slight hallucinations. These reactions are to be expected as the patient attempts to express him- or herself. Some of the emotional links are complicated and will be mentioned in detail later, but the general associations are as follows:

- The Crown chakra is associated with melancholy and several phobias.

- The Brow chakra is associated with anger.
- The Throat chakra is associated with shyness, introversion, and paranoia.
- The Heart chakra is associated with tearfulness, anxiety, depression, and detachedness.
- The Solar Plexus chakra is associated with depression and anxiety.
- The Sacral chakra is associated with envy, jealousy, and lust.
- The Base chakra is associated with insecurity, doubt, and many phobias.

Spiritual

Each major chakra also possesses a "spiritual" connotation. This is purely objective, and depending on the philosophy and culture, a different interpretation will be given. Spiritual relationships to each chakra are the original links with the energy centers, since for centuries they were solely used in meditation and yoga practices. These links are as follows:

- The Crown chakra is coupled with superconsciousness and "all that is."
- The Brow chakra is coupled with intuition.
- The Throat chakra is coupled with expression.
- The Heart chakra is coupled with love.
- The Solar Plexus chakra is coupled with stabilizing control and "Earth."
- The Sacral chakra is coupled with pleasure and enjoyment.
- The Base chakra is coupled with the material and the physical.

Autonomic Nerve Plexus (ANS)

Searching for the relationship between the chakras and the autonomic nervous system has been one of my many research projects over the years. This book explains definitive relationships that are not to be found anywhere else. The links between the endocrine glands and autonomic nervous system are already known, so you do not need to take a huge leap of faith in connecting the chakras to their ANS correspondences. The advent of our ability to analyze through the cranial rhythm has allowed these links to be proven clinically. This relationship is of huge significance in practical therapeutics, since it is now appreciated how important the autonomic nervous system is in the whole sphere of healing. The relationships are as follows:

- The Crown chakra is not linked with the ANS system.
- The Brow chakra is linked with the superior cervical ganglion.
- The Throat chakra is linked with the inferior cervical ganglion.
- The Heart chakra is linked with the celiac plexus and ganglion.
- The Solar Plexus chakra is also linked with the celiac plexus and ganglion.
- The Sacral chakra is linked with the inferior mesenteric ganglion.
- The Base chakra is linked with the Pelvic Plexus. (See Figure 2.3.)

Rotating Vortices

Clairvoyants have reported being able to see several individual rotating vortices within each chakra. Each chakra's vortices are different in color, striations, and number. The number of rotating vortices or petals within the centers reflects the subtlety of each chakra. The lower the number of petals in the chakra, the more "physical" and dense are the relationships and attributed symptoms. The higher the number, the less dense and subtler is the chakra, thus giving a more emotionally related illness, such as depression or anxiety. The number of rotating vortices is unimportant therapeutically when using the chakras in the physical and etheric components of each center. They become more significant when analyzing and healing with the emotional body, where the different components of each chakra will "feel" different, depending on the disease.

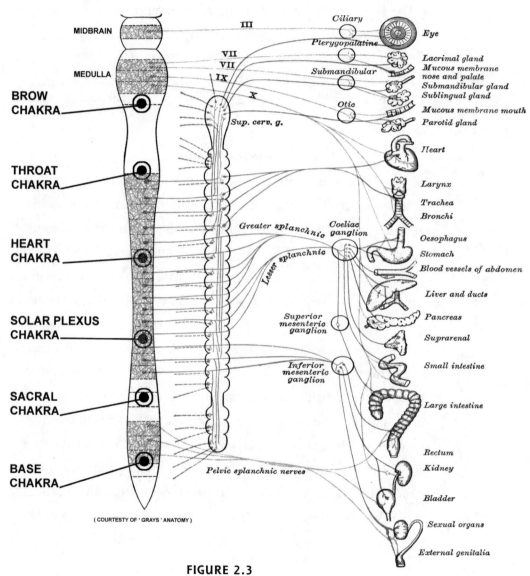

FIGURE 2.3

Associations of the Major Chakras with the Autonomic Nervous System

- The Crown chakra has 972 rotating vortices.
- The Brow chakra has ninety-six rotating vortices.
- The Throat chakra has sixteen rotating vortices.
- The Heart chakra has twelve rotating vortices.
- The Solar Plexus chakra has ten rotating vortices.
- The Sacral chakra has six rotating vortices.
- The Base chakra has four rotating vortices.

See the Color Plates 2–8 for a clairvoyant's interpretation of these vortices.

Sound and Color

As stated many times already, all is energy. This includes sound and color. The particular vibrations at which sound and color resonate are made use of in several types of therapies. Sound and color therapies are, of course, popular in their own right, but when combined with the chakra energies they are made more powerful. Each of these modalities may be used for diagnosis and treatment. Everyone has different sounds and colors that are both harmonizing and jarring. The color a person finds either jarring or harmonizing may indicate that a particular chakra is in a state of imbalance. In treatment mode, a particular sound or color may be transmitted to a particular chakra in healing. You may direct the color itself from a colored lantern or Perspex to the chakra itself, or you may have the patient sit in a room where the color pervades. In sound therapy, the patient is encouraged to recite affirmations or mantras at a certain pitch, which resonate with a particular chakra. The harmonious resonating relationships are as follows:

- The Crown chakra resonates to violet, gold, white and to sound pitch B.
- The Brow chakra resonates to indigo blue and to sound pitch A.

- The Throat chakra resonates to turquoise or sky blue and to sound pitch G.
- The Heart chakra resonates to green and to sound pitch F.
- The Solar Plexus chakra resonates to yellow and to sound pitch E.
- The Sacral chakra resonates to orange and to sound pitch D.
- The Base chakra resonates to red and to sound pitch C.

Vibrational Rate

The vibrational rate represents the numbers used by radionic practitioners when transmitting a "rate" to treat and energy-balance each chakra. They are based on several sources of rates as given in books on radionics and represent the ones that I used when I was a practicing radionic practitioner. Each rate is given in the tables to be found in each section about the major chakras.

Frequency

As explained in the last chapter, the frequency refers to the resonance within each chakra, as scientifically proven. They appear at the end of the tables discussing the individual chakras.

INDIVIDUAL MAJOR CHAKRAS

Let us now turn to the positioning, function, and symptomatology of each of the major chakras.

Chakra 1—Crown—*Sahasrara*
Position

There is only one position for the Crown chakra, at point GOV 20, which is situated on the top of the skull in the very center between the eyebrows and the base of the skull and midway between an imaginary line between the front of each ear. (See Figure 2.4.)

Function

This chakra does not come into full functioning until a person has reached a high level of inner development. It manifests as the pineal

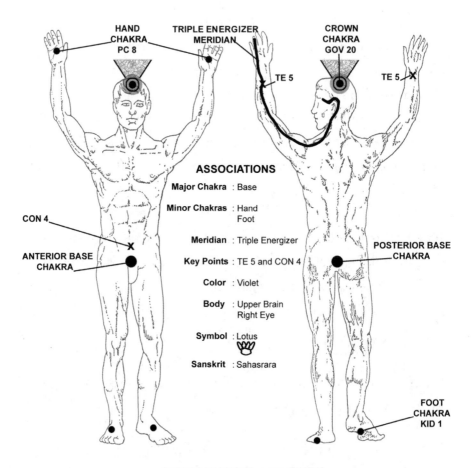

FIGURE 2.4
Associations of the Crown Chakra

gland, which medical science knows is more active in children up to the age of seven but which is thought to then slow down. Research has shown that this gland is connected with visual perception. The gland produces a hormone called melatonin, which regulates the light-reactive photoreceptors in the retina. Continuous light decreases melatonin production, and increased production at night is said to be calming. During the day, the pineal gland produces high levels of another hormone, serotonin, which influences activity. These two hormones work in a continuous circadian cycle. Serotonin has an important influence on our emotional state; high levels of it improve the mood and induce calm. It is for this reason that the chakra is used so much in meditation and yoga.

The Crown chakra, sometimes called the thousand-petaled lotus, is said to govern the upper brain (upper motor neurons) and the right eye. It is also said to be the link between a person and his or her spiritual plane of existence through to the Divine body. This chakra is used extensively in various forms of meditation and yoga. In "spiritual" terms, this chakra is certainly the most important, but probably the least important when used with forms of contact therapy. Therapists should take care when balancing and treating this chakra, since there is a possibility of "detaching" the patient from reality, and he or she may feel lightheaded or "spaced out." This should be a rare occurrence, however, if correct steps are taken. The associated meridian is the Triple Energizer channel, and TE 5 is its main Key point, with Con 4 being the secondary Key point.

Symptoms

Vertigo, tinnitus, high and low blood pressure, right-sided migraines, other types of headache, symptoms of upper-motor neuron disease

TABLE 2.2. THE CROWN CHAKRA

Anatomical position ventral	Top of skull
Anatomical position dorsal	Top of skull
Acupoint ventral	Gov 20
Acupoint dorsal	Gov 20
Sanskrit	*Sahasrara*
Symbol	Lotus
Coupled major chakra	Base
Coupled minor chakras	Hand chakra and Foot chakra
Endocrine gland	Pineal
Associated organs	Upper brain, right eye
Spinal level covered	Cranium
Key point	TE 5
Associated meridian	Triple Energizer
Associated muscles	Trapezius, supraspinatus, facial muscles
Emotions	Melancholy, phobias
Spiritual	Superconsciousness, all that is
Autonomic nerve plexus	None
Number of rotating vortices	972
Sound pitch	B
Associated color	Violet, gold, and white
Vibrational rate (radionics)	6668610.76
Frequency	0.25 hertz

such as multiple sclerosis, Seasonal Affective Disorder (SAD), brittle nails, and lackluster hair.

When the symptoms are obviously opposite in nature, for example, high and low blood pressure, then the chakra may show different forms of energy imbalance. There can be a sluggishness of energy, yielding chronic (yin) symptoms or a hyperactivity of energy that yields acute (yang) symptoms. You will also notice that some conditions and states of imbalance appear in more that one chakra. As you can see from the list of symptoms associated with the Crown chakra, it is not an intensive one, and indeed this chakra is not one that is used in isolation very much, with the possible exception of when a practitioner is treating hypertension and cranial headaches. It is, though, used extensively in combination with other chakras, both major and minor. It can be used in tandem with the Brow center in the treatment of headaches, dizziness, eyestrain, tinnitus, TMJ syndrome, nasal symptoms, and vertigo.

Chakra 2—Brow—*Ajna*
Position

The Brow Chakra is situated at the inion, at the occipital-atlas junction. The acupuncture point is Gov 16. Ventrally it is situated midway between the eyes at point Extra 1 (Yintang). This point is sometimes called Gov 24.5. (See Figure 2.5.)

Function

In esoteric literature, this chakra is said to represent the third eye. This association is very appropriate, since it is most useful in treating conditions of both physical and emotional perception. It is said that extrasensory perception and clairvoyance are externalized through the third eye chakra, and this chakra plays a very important role in intuition. The Brow is said to affect a person's personality, and it externalizes as the pituitary gland, which is the master gland of the endocrine system. If any of the other endocrine glands are not secreting enough of their particular hormone, the pituitary gland will help out by secreting trophic hormone, which often leads to imbalances, such as migraines.

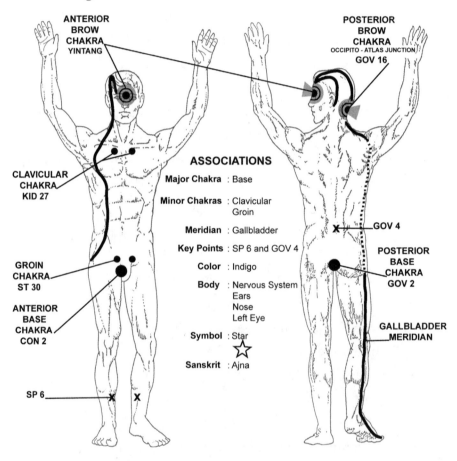

ANTERIOR BROW CHAKRA YINTANG

POSTERIOR BROW CHAKRA OCCIPITO - ATLAS JUNCTION GOV 16

CLAVICULAR CHAKRA KID 27

GROIN CHAKRA ST 30

ANTERIOR BASE CHAKRA CON 2

SP 6

GOV 4

POSTERIOR BASE CHAKRA GOV 2

GALLBLADDER MERIDIAN

ASSOCIATIONS

Major Chakra : Base

Minor Chakras : Clavicular
                Groin

Meridian : Gallbladder

Key Points : SP 6 and GOV 4

Color : Indigo

Body : Nervous System
       Ears
       Nose
       Left Eye

Symbol : Star ☆

Sanskrit : Ajna

INTUITION : INTELLECTUAL

FIGURE 2.5
Associations of the Brow Chakra

TABLE 2.3. THE BROW CHAKRA

Anatomical position ventral	Between the eyes
Anatomical position dorsal	Atlanto-occipital junction (inion)
Acupoint point ventral	Yintang (Extra 1) or Gov 24.5
Acupoint point dorsal	Gov 16
Sanskrit	*Ajna*
Symbol	Star
Coupled major chakra	Base
Coupled minor chakras	Clavicular and Groin
Endocrine gland	Pituitary
Associated organs	Lower brain, nervous system, ears, nose, left eye
Spinal level governed	Cranial base—C 4
Key point	SP 6
Associated meridian	Gallbladder
Associated muscles	Anterior and posterior neck muscles
Emotions	Anger
Spiritual	Intuition, intellect
Autonomic nerve plexus	Ciliary ganglion
Number of rotating vortices	Ninety-six
Sound pitch	A
Associate color	Indigo
Vibrational rate (radionics)	66674789
Frequency	2.96 hertz

Many texts incorrectly associate the Brow center with the pineal gland and the Crown with the pituitary. The reason is that the Brow is associated with the "secret" eye and not with sight as such. The Brow, through the pituitary and hypothalamus, is concerned with intuitional sight. When you use acupuncture to influence the Brow center, it has significant influences on hormonal secretions (via the pituitary); this would be impossible to bring about by using the Crown center. It is possible to do this with acupressure, but it is a long process, albeit a rewarding one. The Brow center governs the lower brain (the brain stem and cerebellum), the left eye, the nose, the ears, and the central nervous system. It is an extremely important chakra when used in combination with other chakras and acupoints for the control of hormones. The Brow chakra at acupoint Extra 1 (Yintang) is the equivalent of acupoint Bladder 1 and shares many of its functions. The chakra's Key points are SP 6 and Gov 4, and it is associated with the Gallbladder meridian.

Symptoms

Migraine, chronic and acute catarrh, sinusitis, infectious and contagious disease, deafness and altered hearing, arthritis of the upper cervical spine, TMJ syndrome, Ménière's disease, vertigo, dizziness and lightheadedness, headaches, stress and worry, some motor neuron disease symptoms, rage, and shyness.

It is in the treatment of catarrh, sinusitis, and conditions affecting the eustachian tube that this very powerful center has its best use within acupressure and acupuncture. It is also the focal point in the treatment of the symptoms of many upper- and lower-motor neuron ailments such as multiple sclerosis, Parkinson's disease, and ataxia. As with all the dual-based chakras, the dorsal aspect helps with the treatment of musculoskeletal conditions, and the ventral aspect best addresses organic and neurological conditions. The two aspects of the chakra are probably the most powerful antistress and relaxation duo of points in the whole body. Balancing their energy can yield very rewarding results.

Chakra 3—Throat—*Vishuddha*
Position

The Throat or *Vishuddha* chakra is situated at the junction of the seventh cervical and the first thoracic vertebra (C7-T1) at the base of the neck. The acupoint is Gov 14. The ventral aspect is at point Con 22 at the center of the sternal notch. (See Figure 2.6.)

Function

This is a very powerful chakra. It is probably the second most commonly used chakra, next to the Base chakra. The Throat chakra is said to be the lowest chakra of the higher self and manifests physically through the thyroid and parathyroid glands. It often becomes congested when dealing with invading organisms and viruses that produce the physical symptoms of sore throats and tonsillitis. It tends, therefore, to be the body's first line of defense. It is useful in treating acute febrile disease caused by bacteria and viruses. This chakra is also useful in treating the long-term effects of the suppression of these glands by drug therapy that may be a contributing factor in glandular fever and asthma. It is said to be in a state of imbalance in people who cannot express themselves easily or in those who are reclusive, shy, or introverted. Damage to this chakra may be caused by sudden emotional shock such as grief.

This chakra is very much concerned with *excretion* at all levels. It is associated with the large bowel and lungs, both of which pertain to physical excretion. It is also concerned with the excretion of wasteful thoughts and "hang-ups" (which are not the same as phobias). Its association with the minor chakras of the Shoulder and Navel underline this influence on excretion processes. When a patient shows a state of congestion either at a physical or emotional level, the Throat chakra must be balanced and treated. Often, when he or she has

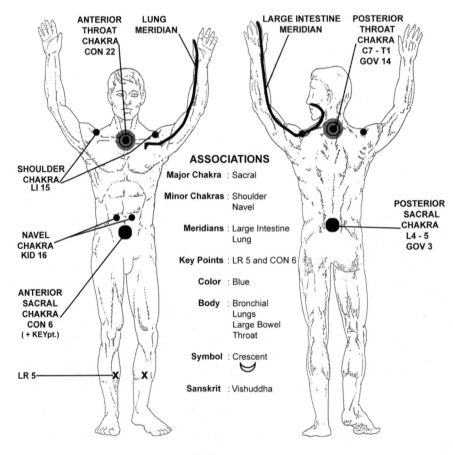

ANTERIOR THROAT CHAKRA CON 22

LUNG MERIDIAN

LARGE INTESTINE MERIDIAN

POSTERIOR THROAT CHAKRA C7 - T1 GOV 14

SHOULDER CHAKRA LI 15

NAVEL CHAKRA KID 16

ANTERIOR SACRAL CHAKRA CON 6 (+ KEYpt.)

LR 5   X   X

POSTERIOR SACRAL CHAKRA L4 - 5 GOV 3

ASSOCIATIONS

Major Chakra : Sacral

Minor Chakras : Shoulder
Navel

Meridians : Large Intestine
Lung

Key Points : LR 5 and CON 6

Color : Blue

Body : Bronchial
Lungs
Large Bowel
Throat

Symbol : Crescent

Sanskrit : Vishuddha

EXPRESSION : EXCRETION

FIGURE 2.6
Associations of the Throat Chakra

TABLE 2.4. THE THROAT CHAKRA

Anatomical position ventral	Sternal notch
Anatomical position dorsal	C7-T1
Acupuncture point ventral	Con 22
Acupuncture point dorsal	Gov 14
Sanskrit	*Vishuddha*
Symbol	Crescent
Coupled major chakra	Sacral
Coupled minor chakras	Shoulder and navel
Endocrine glands	Thyroid and parathyroid
Associated organs	Bronchial tubes, lungs, vocal cords, alimentary tract, throat, skin
Spinal level covered	C5-T3
Key points	LR 5 and Con 6
Associated meridians	Large intestine and lung
Associated muscles	Latissimus dorsi, pectorals, triceps,
Emotions	Forearm muscles
Spiritual	Shyness, introversion, paranoia
Autonomic nerve plexus	Expression
Number of rotating vortices	Superior cervical ganglion
Sound	Sixteen
Pitch	G
Associated color	Blue
Vibrational rate (radionics)	66678575
Frequency	81.2 hertz

experienced old emotions or throat congestion, the patient will have a sensation of gagging when the therapist's hand is placed, even gently, over the throat area. This is a good indicator that the chakra needs treatment. The esoteric texts will suggest that yoga or meditation be performed to clear the chakra, but very useful hands-on therapy or acupuncture can also be used to clear congestion. The Key points are LR 5 (found two cun, or three fingers width, superior to SP 6 on the medial aspect of the tibia) and Con 6. (A cun is sometimes called a "Chinese inch" and is equivalent to the width of the thumb.) The associated meridians are the Large Intestine and the Lung.

Symptoms

Migraine, acute and chronic sore throats, tonsillitis, asthma, loss of taste, acute and chronic bronchitis and other respiratory tract infections, laryngitis, colitis and irritable bowel syndrome, ileocaecal valve syndrome, chronic skin lesions such as eczema and alopecia, shyness, introversion, and paranoia.

The posterior aspect of this chakra, situated at the cervico-thoracic junction, is very useful in the treatment of stress that culminates in tension of the neck muscles, fibrositis, and some types of frozen shoulder. Chelation (massage) around and away from the area can be beneficial in cases of soft tissue congestion and fibrositis.

Chakra 4—Heart—*Anahata*
Position

The Heart, or *Anahata,* chakra is situated at the center of the thoracic spine at level T6-T7. The acupuncture point is Gov 10. The ventral aspect is situated halfway down the sternum at Con 17. (See Figure 2.7.)

Function

If the Throat chakra is one of the most used centers, the Heart chakra is one of the least used in clinical therapy concerning physical ailments. Its great significance is in the treatment of emotional imbalance. The glandular counterpart of this chakra is the thymus, which is involved in the autoimmune system. When this chakra is over-

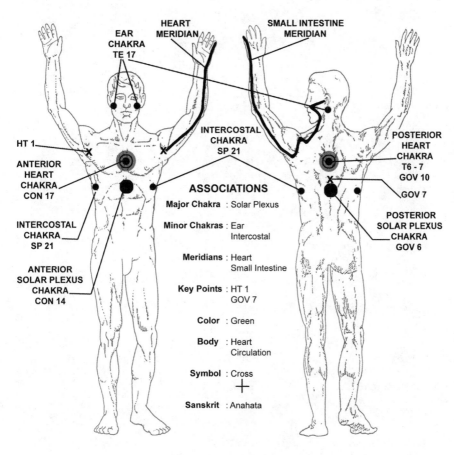

ANXIETY : DETACHMENT : LOVE

FIGURE 2.7
Associations of the Heart Chakra

TABLE 2.5. THE HEART CHAKRA

Anatomical position	Ventral midsternum
Anatomical position	Dorsal T6-T7
Acupuncture point	Ventral Con 17
Acupuncture point	Dorsal Gov 10
Sanskrit	*Anahata*
Symbol	Cross
Coupled major chakra	Solar plexus
Coupled minor chakras	Ear and Intercostal
Endocrine gland	Thymus
Associated organs	Heart, veins and arteries, vagus nerve
Spinal level covered	T4-T8
Key points	HT 1 and Gov 7
Associated meridians	Heart and small intestine
Associated muscles	Erector spinae
Emotions	Tearfulness, anxiety
Spiritual	Love
Autonomic nerve plexus	Inferior cervical ganglion
Number of rotating vortices	Twelve
Sound pitch	F
Associated color	Green
Vibrational rate (radionics)	66664424
Frequency	7.8 hertz

active, it can produce amoral, irresponsible behavior. Energy flooding uncontrolled into this center can have a devastating effect on the personality of the person, especially in affairs of the heart! Over-stimulation can produce a state of sheer bliss, such as what one feels when falling in love, almost producing an "out-of-this-world" feeling. People easily cry and become upset. This is the chakra of the "giggler" and of those who weep when telling their sorrowful stories at consultation. Executives and tycoons have great strain put on their Heart chakras and can suffer heart trouble as a consequence. Doctors and therapists who cannot detach themselves from their patients are in a similar plight (therapists, please take note!). Thoracic scoliosis is a common condition treated via this chakra if it is not too chronic and fused. The associated meridians are Heart and Small Intestine, and the Key points are HT 1 and Gov 7.

Symptoms

Benign tumors and growths, scoliosis, heart conditions ranging from congestive heart failure to simple circulatory imbalance, palpitation, angina, varicosities, tearfulness, anxiety, insularity, and introversion.

Some care should be taken when initially balancing this center anteriorly and posteriorly (to be discussed in a later chapter), since the patient could be prone to fainting if he or she is sitting up and has a history of emotional imbalance. Please have the patient lie down on his or her side; it makes life a lot easier.

Chakra 5—Solar Plexus—*Manipura*
Position

The Solar Plexus chakra is situated at the junction of the thoracic and lumbar spine at T12-L1. The acupuncture point there is Gov 6.

The ventral aspect is located just below the xiphoid process of the sternum at Con 14. (See Figure 2.8.)

Function

This chakra represents a vast clearinghouse of energies found below the diaphragm. In most people it is active, either congested or over-stimulated, caused by eating foods with additives or denatured foods,

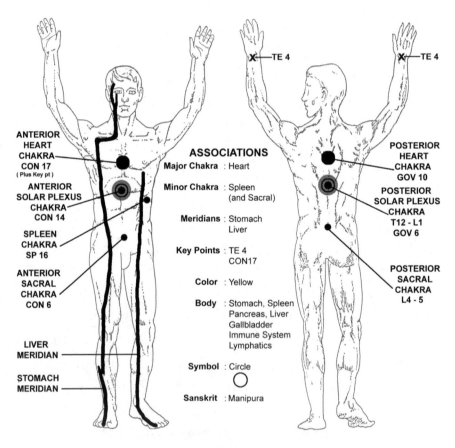

ANTERIOR
HEART
CHAKRA
CON 17
(Plus Key pt)

ANTERIOR
SOLAR PLEXUS
CHAKRA
CON 14

SPLEEN
CHAKRA
SP 16

ANTERIOR
SACRAL
CHAKRA
CON 6

LIVER
MERIDIAN

STOMACH
MERIDIAN

TE 4
TE 4

POSTERIOR
HEART
CHAKRA
GOV 10

POSTERIOR
SOLAR PLEXUS
CHAKRA
T12 - L1
GOV 6

POSTERIOR
SACRAL
CHAKRA
L4 - 5

ASSOCIATIONS

Major Chakra : Heart

Minor Chakra : Spleen
(and Sacral)

Meridians : Stomach
Liver

Key Points : TE 4
CON17

Color : Yellow

Body : Stomach, Spleen
Pancreas, Liver
Gallbladder
Immune System
Lymphatics

Symbol : Circle

○

Sanskrit : Manipura

STABILISING : CONTROL : EARTH

FIGURE 2.8
Associations of the Solar Plexus Chakra

TABLE 2.6. THE SOLAR PLEXUS CHAKRA

Anatomical position ventral	Below the xiphoid process of the sternum
Anatomical position dorsal	T12-L1
Acupuncture point ventral	Con 14
Acupuncture point dorsal	Gov 6
Sanskrit	*Manipura*
Symbol	Circle
Coupled major chakra	Heart
Coupled minor chakra	Spleen
Endocrine gland	Pancreas
Associated organs	Stomach, liver, spleen, pancreas, duodenum, gallbladder
Spinal area covered	T9-L2
Key points	TE 4 and Con 17
Associated meridians	Liver and Stomach
Associated muscles	Abdominals, quadriceps
Emotions	Depression, worry, anxiety
Spiritual	Stabilizing, control, Earth
Autonomic nerve plexus	Celiac plexus and ganglion
Number of rotating vortices	Ten
Sound pitch	E
Associated color	Yellow
Vibrational rate (radionics)	6666410.53
Frequency	23.0 hertz

or by the sheer pace of life. This can result in nervous disorders and stomach, liver, gallbladder, pancreas, and spleen disease. If the imbalance becomes chronic, this can give rise to a decrease in the energy potential of the body's immune system and create conditions such as chronic fatigue syndrome (CFS). Weakness in this area due to a congested chakra can cause scoliosis or muscular imbalance. This may further affect the cervical and lumbar spine as they attempt to compensate for the midthoracic misalignments. The Solar Plexus chakra is vitally important, therefore, in the treatment of many organic and emotional conditions. It is always important to balance the energies of the Heart chakra to that of the Solar Plexus before treatment commences, since the emotional symptoms and the etiology are very similar and obviously connected. The associated endocrine gland is the pancreas, which produces insulin and is involved in the metabolism of sugar. The associated meridians are the Liver and Stomach, and the Key points are TE 4 and Con 17.

Symptoms

Skin conditions such as eczema and acne, stomach ulcers, cancerous growths, hepatitis, gallbladder colic, indigestion and dyspepsia, infections of the glandular system as a whole, glandular fever, chronic fatigue syndrome, allergies, hay fever, small intestine spasms, irritable bowel syndrome, ileocaecal valve syndrome, worry, depression, and anxiety.

The main two chronic illnesses associated with imbalance in the Solar Plexux chakra are diabetes and cancer. Although these diseases often have physical and chemical causes, symptoms are often precipitated by an imbalance in the mental and emotional bodies. Diabetes may be caused by a person not allowing enough sweetness and love to enter his or her life, and holding onto the emotions of anger, fear, and hatred may be a contributing cause of cancer. Conventional medical treatment often works extremely well (and obviously saves lives), but it does not treat the root cause of the situation. It is imperative to instruct the patient in meditation or yoga as well as in receiving their treatment via the chakras. They may do these things at the done at the same time that they receive their more conventional treatments. The solar plexus is often called the seat of our emotions. The phrase "having a gut feeling" about matters concerns the solar plexus. Having "butterflies" in the stomach in times of stress or just before an important event also indicate an overactive Solar Plexus chakra. These symptoms disappear when the patent relaxes (except in cases of chronic thoracic inflammation, which may be sending referred pain to the stomach and diaphragmatic region).

Chakra 6—Sacral—*Svadhisthana*
Position

The Sacral chakra is situated at the junction of lumbar 4-5 near the base of the spine. The acupuncture point there is Gov 3. The ventral aspect is at Con 6, which is located 1.5 cun (two finger widths) below the umbilicus. This frontal point is also called the *hara*, a point that is widely used in meditative practices and yoga, as well as in martial arts and subtle energy movements such as aikido and tai chi. (See Figure 2.9.)

Function

This chakra is said to rule both the reproductive system and the control of water within the body. It is used extensively in conditions related to these systems. It is also coupled with the Throat chakra, and the two make an excellent couple in the treatment of edema and chronic sore throats, among many other conditions. In combination with the Base chakra, it is also used in the treatment of lumbar spine, sacral, and sacroiliac conditions. It is, however, its use in reproductive, gynecological, and obstetric conditions that is most extensive. In some texts, this chakra is known as the Spleen or Navel chakra.

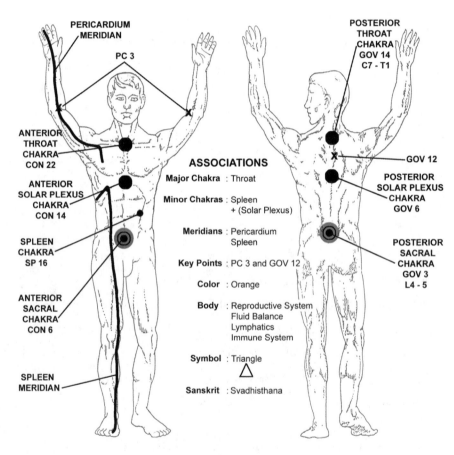

ASSOCIATIONS

Major Chakra	: Throat
Minor Chakras	: Spleen + (Solar Plexus)
Meridians	: Pericardium Spleen
Key Points	: PC 3 and GOV 12
Color	: Orange
Body	: Reproductive System Fluid Balance Lymphatics Immune System
Symbol	: Triangle △
Sanskrit	: Svadhisthana

PLEASURE : ENJOYMENT : SEXUAL

FIGURE 2.9

Associations of the Sacral Chakra

TABLE 2.7. THE SACRAL CHAKRA

Anatomical position ventral	Just below the navel *(hara)*
Anatomical position dorsal	L4-5
Acupuncture point ventral	Con 6
Acupuncture point dorsal	Gov 3
Sanskrit	*Svadisthana*
Symbol	Triangle
Coupled major chakra	Throat
Coupled minor chakra	Spleen
Endocrine glands	Gonads and uterus
Associated organs	Reproductive system, fluid balance, lymphatics
Spinal level covered	L2-S2
Key points	PC 3 and Gov 12
Associated meridians	Spleen and Pericardium
Associated muscles	Hamstrings, anterior and posterior tibials
Emotions	Jealousy, envy, lust
Spiritual	Pleasure, enjoyment, relationships
Autonomic nerve plexus	Inferior mesenteric ganglion
Number of rotating vortices	Six
Sound pitch	D
Associated color	Orange
Vibration rate (radionics)	66663206
Frequency	81.1 hertz

My research and practice dispute this. These two are minor chakras in their own right with separate functions.

The Sacral chakra is also associated with the lower third of the small intestine, hence its involvement in the area of assimilation. With water control in the body, there is obviously an effect on the kidneys, but there does not appear to be a strong influence on the Sacral chakra. In my opinion, the kidneys are associated with the Base chakra. It cannot be denied, though, that a Sacral chakra imbalance affects water rhythms within the body. Certain Native American shamanic teachings associate all water creatures with the Sacral chakra. The lunar cycle also has a huge influence on our water system cycle. Other circadian and monthly cycles, including the menstrual cycle, are governed by this chakra.

Some texts link this chakra with the adrenals. Yet extensive research and clinical practice on my part has shown that the endocrine link is to the uterus and gonads, not to the adrenals. If this chakra is underactive, the patient has an urge to eat excessively. He or she will also experience an increased sex drive. These factors may cause obesity, food intolerance, chronic skin conditions, and possibly impotence. Traditional teaching tells us to regain Sacral (sacred) equilibrium through dance, some good belly laughs), yoga, breathing exercises, and visualizing orange light. The associated meridians are the Spleen and Pericardium, and the Key points are PC 3 and Gov 12.

Symptoms

Low vitality, intestinal and gastric conditions, irritable bowel syndrome, chronic tiredness and lethargy, impotence, unusually high or low libido, chronic sore throat, imbalance with the heating mechanism, including cold feet and chilblains, menstrual and menopausal conditions, edema, swollen ankles, and some rheumatoid factor conditions.

Chakra 7—Base—*Muladhara*
Position

The Base chakra is situated at the base of the spine at the sacrococcygeal junction at point Gov 2. The ventral aspect is on the upper crest of the symphysis pubis at Con 2. The positions given are those for performing hands-on therapy. The exact position of the chakra is below the coccyx and at the perineum. There is really just *one* physical counterpart position. It is obvious, though, that in the practical treatment of this highly important chakra, it needs to be "acceptable" to touch therapy. There is, of course, an area of influence that affects the chakra when working at Gov 2 and Con 2. The Base chakra is used more than any other chakra in all types of conditions. Always warn you patient before placing your hand on that part of his or her anatomy. (See Figure 2.10.)

Function

As stated above, the Base chakra (sometimes called the Root chakra) is probably used more than any other chakra in everyday clinical work. It is used to treat any *chronic* condition. In isolation and in combination with other relevant chakras, it is used to treat chronic mechanical, osteoarthritic, hereditary, and deep emotional conditions. The Base chakra is said to be responsible for anchoring the body on the physical plane and providing a channel for the will to express itself. Although, it is said to be relatively inactive and dormant in the general population, its activity is on the increase owing to the stress of modern living.

It is associated with the adrenal medulla and cortex, the former being responsible for the production of adrenaline and the latter of cortisone. This is the chakra used in the treatment of deep-seated hereditary and miasmatic weakness. It is the focal point for any problem or condition concerning the spinal column and the kidneys. Psychosomatic problems, such as the will to live being at a low ebb, are also associated with this chakra.

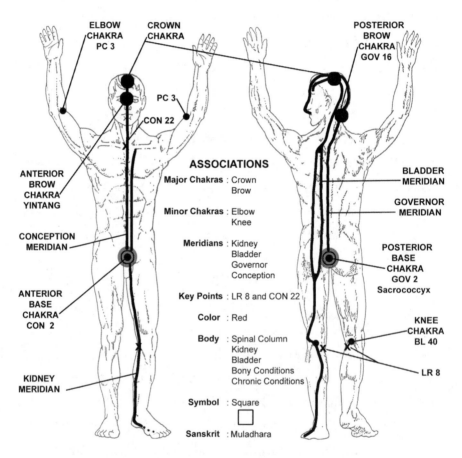

ASSOCIATIONS

Major Chakras : Crown
Brow

Minor Chakras : Elbow
Knee

Meridians : Kidney
Bladder
Governor
Conception

Key Points : LR 8 and CON 22

Color : Red

Body : Spinal Column
Kidney
Bladder
Bony Conditions
Chronic Conditions

Symbol : Square

Sanskrit : Muladhara

MATERIAL : PHYSICAL : GROUNDING : ANCESTRY

FIGURE 2.10
Associations of the Base Chakra

TABLE 2.8. THE BASE CHAKRA

Anatomical position ventral	Symphysis pubis
Anatomical position dorsal	Sacrococcyx junction
Acupuncture point ventral	Con 2
Acupuncture point dorsal	Gov 2
Sanskrit	*Muladhara*
Symbol	Square
Coupled major chakras	Crown and Brow
Coupled minor chakras	Elbow and Knee
Endocrine gland	Adrenals
Associated organs	Spinal column, kidneys, bladder, ureter
Spinal level covered	S3 to tip of coccyx
Key points	LR 8 and Con 22
Associated meridians	Bladder and Kidney
Associated muscles	Psoas/Iliacus, soleus, gastrocnemius, foot muscles
Emotions	Insecurity, doubt
Spiritual	Material and physical
Autonomic nerve plexus	Pelvic plexus
Number of rotating vortices	Four
Sound pitch	C
Associated color	Red
Vibrational rate (radionics)	66658874
Frequency	81.1 hertz

In his book *Radionics and the Subtle Anatomy of Man*, David Tansley writes:

> Premature overstimulation of the Base chakra can result in the burning away of the protective etheric webs along the spine, thus opening the chakras to forces that the individual is not yet capable of handling. Those who foolishly spend their time trying to open up the chakras by meditating upon them or attempting to arouse the kundalini in an effort to take a spiritual short cut that does not in reality exist, are courting danger. Fortunately, most people who dabble in certain forms of yoga and meditation are protected by their own gross ignorance of the subject. The substance of the physical body is animated by the Base chakra. The kundalini energies, when aroused correctly and controlled in full consciousness, progress up the spine in a geometric pattern similar to the snakes of the Caduceus, symbol of the healing arts. Curiously enough, the same pattern is also seen in the double helix configuration of the DNA molecules, containing the code of life. Perhaps this too reflects the connection between the Base chakra and the cellular substance of the physical body.

Please do not be concerned about raising the kundalini in the everyday practice of working with the chakra energy system—it will not happen! To raise kundalini energy takes months, if not years, of constant meditation and centering practice. Use the Base chakra constantly without being hindered by any of these worries. It is one thing to use the chakras in meditation over the years and quite another to use them with physical therapy in the short term. The Base chakra represents an extremely powerful region that can be used in healing. It is the influence of the Base chakra that tends to keep us earthbound. We all need "roots" and to be grounded. The associated meridians are the Kidney and Bladder, and the Key points are LR 8 and Con 22.

Symptoms

Osteoarthritis, ankylosing spondylitis, rheumatoid arthritis, stiff joints, nephritis, chronic cystitis, chronic and acute prostatitis, gravitational ulcers, "growing" pains, Scheurmann's disease; other bone diseases, such as Osgood Sclatter's syndrome; depression, lethargy, and chronic tiredness; chronic pelvic, sacral, lumbar, thoracic, cervical, and cranial conditions; some phobias, and insanity.

Now that we have explored the individual major chakras, let us turn to the minor chakras. There is much more to say about the major chakras, and indeed, many more details about them can be found in other books. As stated before, most other books on the topic deal with yoga practices, meditation, and esoteric physiology. Although all the information is important, this book is for the practicing therapist and therefore includes descriptions that are down-to-earth and pertinent to clinical therapy.

THE TWENTY-ONE MINOR CHAKRAS

As of this writing, there are no books that discuss the minor chakras in depth. So far I have read just three books in which they are given a mention, and two of them are based on Tansley's original diagram of their positioning (see *Radionics and the Subtle Anatomy of Man*). Most of the positions that are given in that book are, in my opinion, incorrect. I have undertaken several years' research as to their location and function, and the information provided below is original and unique in its concept and practice.

Why are they called minor chakras, and why are there said to be twenty-one of them? They are called minor because they are inferior in energy to the major chakras but much more powerful than most "ordinary" acupoints. I count twenty-one because there are ten bilateral points, plus the odd one—the Spleen chakra. Earlier I stated that each point on the physical body is a gateway to the astral plane (our higher selves) and that each point represents the thirteen (six are bilateral) most powerful points on the body. Clairvoyants have told us that each major chakra has twenty-one concentric circles or whorls of energy. They also tell us that the minor chakras are the second most important sets of acupoints/triggers/energy points on the body because they are said to have fourteen concentric circles of energy. The major acupoints such as LI 4, LR 3, and so on have seven concentric whorls, and the minor acupoints and reflex points have between two and five, depending on their importance. All this represents a field that needs to be investigated.

In playing the devil's advocate though, I cannot totally buy in to this theory. It just seems too vague. I have chosen the points representing the physical components of the minor chakras through common sense (hopefully) and practical research. Although the minor chakras are powerful energy points in their own right, there is no evidence of astral or spiritual connections except to the emotional limit of the etheric body. They can therefore be considered to be reflex points or reflected pathways of the seven majors chakras. Their main characteristic that has been proved beyond a doubt is their use in *pain relief*. They also have many other functions, which will be mentioned in the next chapter.

Positions

The numbering and positions of the minor chakras are as follows (see Figure 2.1):

1. Spleen chakra located at left SP 16.

2 and 3. Foot chakra located at KID 1 bilateral.

4 and 5. Hand chakra located at PC 8 bilateral.

6 and 7. Knee chakra located at BL 40 bilateral.

8 and 9. Elbow chakra located at PC 3 bilateral.

10 and 11. Groin chakra located at ST 30 bilateral.

12 and 13. Clavicular chakra located at KID 27 bilateral.

14 and 15. Shoulder chakra located at LI 15 bilateral.

16 and 17. Navel chakra located at KID 16 bilateral.

18 and 19. Ear chakra located at TE 17 bilateral.

20 and 21. Intercostal chakra located at SP 21 bilateral.

I have assigned each of the minor chakras my own simple nomenclature. Having read through the esoteric scripts, I have found a Sanskrit translation assigned to each that is similar to the properties of the physical acupoints, but a single Sanskrit word does not exist. It should be noted that apart from the Spleen chakra, all are bilateral points and appear mostly on the anterolateral aspects of the body. Some texts insist that the Spleen chakra is powerful enough (indeed, it is sometimes called the eighth major and often confused with the Sacral chakra) to have two points of contact, one dorsal and one ventral, as do the majors. Although one could argue that the Spleen chakra possesses a dorsal aspect, the one that is used constantly is the left SP 16 point.

It should also be pointed out that each of the acupoints constituting the physical counterpart of each minor chakra is a powerful point in its own right. The reason is obvious—because of the chakra involvement where power and energy are supreme, these acupoints may be adjusted and manipulated in incredible ways. Notice also that three of the minor chakras are situated on the Kidney meridian, and two on the Pericardium. These energies are considered to be the deepest, according to the Six Chious of Traditional Chinese Medicine.

As with the seven major chakras, the twenty bilateral minor chakras each have a coupled minor chakra on the same side of the body, for example, right with right and left with left. This means that when one of the chakras is in a state of imbalance, it can draw energy reserves from its coupled chakra as well as from its "partner" on the same point on the other side of the body. Also, with each minor center, a Key point is used to "open up" the energy flow prior to treatment. Each of the minors has its own associated meridian, symptoms, color, sound pitch, major chakra link, frequency, and vibrational rate used in radionics. The resonance of each minor chakra has also been linked with its own homeopathic remedy, since they appear to have the same frequency. Once again, this is an area of research that could be fruitful. There is also a time of day when energy may be influenced more than at any other time, similar to the Chinese Clock theory, which states that there is an emphasis of chi in a specific organ over a two-hour cycle. This can be of use clinically.

The coupling of the minor chakras needs to be explained in detail. It has been known for centuries, in traditional medicine, that the foot is associated with the hand, and the elbow with the knee, through the so-called parallel areas. Reflexology philosophy has shown that the points and areas on the hands and feet can be used to affect the same organs or parts of the body, as can those on the knees and elbows. The Groin/Clavicular couple lies on the same meridial and zonal line, and both are associated with the Ren Mai (Conception) meridian and the deep ancestral energies of the body. The Ear/Intercostal coupling is situated on the most lateral side of the body in the same zonal line. The Shoulder/Navel couple is associated with elimination of waste from the body—together these chakras make a very powerful pairing. It should also be noted that each minor chakra has one associated meridian, with the exception of the Spleen chakra, which has two.

These coupled meridians seem to be close to the couple that exists within the Six Chious of Traditional Chinese Medicine (TCM). Some traditional texts state that the meridians are one continuous energy loop that flows from hand to foot and from the foot to the hand via the chest. This system of TCM is commonplace in Germany and in some other parts of Europe. In acupressure, instead of the meridian being stroked along a single line, the double meridian is stroked in one continuous movement.

The Key points, with the exception of that of the Spleen chakra, are placed on the coupled meridian, so they should be easy to remember once you learn the meridian. It took an inordinately long time to work out the Key points; there is no easy pattern in learning them. There are a few *luo* points, a couple of tonification points, and a few source points, as well as some more obscure points. You just need to learn them.

Spleen Chakra

The Spleen chakra, said to be the most major chakra among the minors, is the odd one out in every respect. It is closely associated with the Solar Plexus and Sacral chakras, and thus the full benefit of treatment and balancing the energy of this chakra is best obtained when using it in a combination with them. It will be noted that the Spleen chakra at SP 16 (left) and its Key point at Gov 8 are situated along the same horizontal body line. (See Figure 2.11.)

Symptoms

The Spleen chakra follows both conventional and TCM theory when it comes to symptoms caused by energy imbalance:

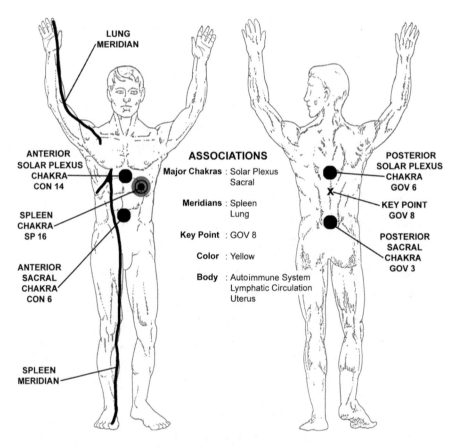

THERE ARE NO PAIN-RELIEF AREAS

FIGURE 2.11
Associations of the Spleen Chakra

1. Autoimmune system
2. Leukocyte imbalance
3. Infection
4. Lymphatic circulation and obstruction
5. Uterine imbalance

The following named conditions can therefore be caused by a Spleen chakra imbalance either in isolation or in combination with its coupled majors of Solar Plexus and Sacral chakras: glandular fever, children's skin conditions, chronic tonsillitis, breast tumors, premenstrual irregularities, leucorrhoea, menopausal symptoms, edema, chronic fatigue syndrome, lethargy, general allergic conditions, hay fever, gravitational ulcers, thoracic scoliosis, and viral infections.

Coupled minor chakra	None
Coupled major chakras	Solar Plexus and Sacral
Meridians	Spleen and Lung
Acupuncture point location	SP 16 (L)
Key point	Gov 8
Time of maximum energy	6:00–10:00 p.m.
Color	Yellow
Sound pitch	E
Vibrational rate (radionics)	445664
Homeopathic remedy	*Carduus marianus*

Let us now turn to the remaining twenty minor chakras. Their main role is in providing pain relief, the practicalities of which are discussed in other chapters; but for now we will explore the many associations, as well as local and general symptoms. Treatment of the symptoms described use the chakra together with either an associated chakra or with other acupoints. It is rare to treat symptoms with just one chakra, major or minor. Although each minor chakra

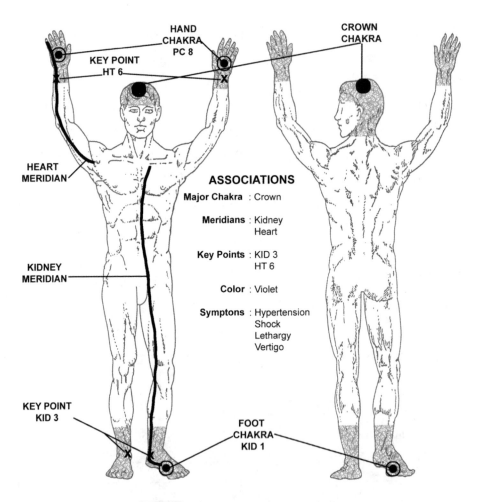

FIGURE 2.12

Associations of the Foot and Hand Chakras

will be described as an entity, the best way to use them is as a pair or trio with its associated chakras.

Foot Chakra

The Foot chakra is situated at KID 1, which is the only meridian acupoint on the sole of the foot. It is a very powerful point, being linked with the Hand and Crown chakras. (See Figure 2.12.)

Local Symptoms

Metatarsalgia, foot pain, dropped arches, callus formation, edema of the foot, heel spurs.

General Symptoms

Hypertension, infantile convulsions, epilepsy, coma, shock, lethargy, dizziness, headaches, migraines, and insomnia.

Coupled minor chakra	Hand
Coupled major chakra	Crown
Meridian	Kidney
Acupoint location	KID 1 (Sole of foot)
Time of maximum energy	12:00–2:00 p.m.
Key point	HT 6
Color	Violet
Sound pitch	B
Vibrational rate (radionics)	111038
Homeopathic remedy	*Silica*

Hand Chakra

The Hand chakra is positioned in the center of the palm at PC 8 (often called the stigmata point; see Figure 2.12).

Local Symptoms

Plantar fasciitis, duputrens contracture, and skin infections local to the hands and nails.

General Symptoms

See the symptoms listed under Foot chakra.

Coupled minor chakra	Foot
Coupled major chakra	Crown
Meridian	Heart
Acupoint location	PC 8 (center of palm)
Key point	KID 3
Time of maximum energy	10:00 a.m.–12:00 p.m.
Color	Violet
Sound pitch	B
Vibrational rate in radionics	996835
Homeopathic remedy	*Thuja*

Knee Chakra

The Knee chakra is positioned in the center of the popliteal fossa. It is associated with the Elbow and Base chakras. (See Figure 2.13.)

Local Symptoms

Sciatica, bursitis, popliteus and posterior knee weakness and discomfort, Osgood Schlatter syndrome, and osteoarthritic changes of the knee, especially at the lateral border.

General Symptoms

Cold feet, poor leg circulation, hip pain, cystitis, sacral sacroiliac pain and joint changes, lumbar spine pain and joint changes, stiff hips.

Coupled minor chakra	Elbow
Coupled major chakra	Base
Meridian	Bladder
Acupoint location	BL 40 (center of popliteal fossa)
Key point	SI 7
Time of energy	2:00–4:00 p.m.
Color	Red
Sound pitch	C
Vibration rate (radionics)	443002
Homeopathic remedy	*Lobelia inflata*

Elbow Chakra

The Elbow chakra is situated in the center of the cubital fossa on the anterior aspect of the elbow at point PC 3 (see Figure 2.13).

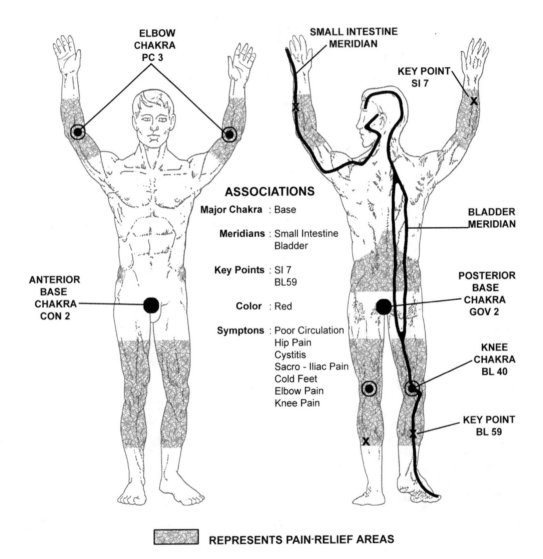

ASSOCIATIONS

Major Chakra	: Base
Meridians	: Small Intestine Bladder
Key Points	: SI 7 BL59
Color	: Red
Symptons	: Poor Circulation Hip Pain Cystitis Sacro - Iliac Pain Cold Feet Elbow Pain Knee Pain

REPRESENTS PAIN-RELIEF AREAS

FIGURE 2.13

Associations of the Knee and Elbow Chakras

Local Symptoms

Elbow joint pain and stiffness with or without joint changes and acute and chronic tennis and golfer's elbow of a nontraumatic etiology.

General Symptoms

These are the same as the symptoms associated with the Knee chakra, with the addition of palpitation and angina.

Coupled minor chakra	Knee
Coupled major chakra	Base
Meridian	Small Intestine
Acupoint location	PC 3 (center of elbow)
Key point	BL 59
Time of maximum energy	4:00–6:00 p.m.
Color	Red
Sound pitch	C
Vibrational rate (radionics)	997436
Homeopathic remedy	*Cactus*

Groin Chakra

This chakra is positioned close to the symphysis pubis at point ST 30. It is associated with the Clavicular and Brow chakras. (See Figure 2.14.)

Local Symptoms

Hip pain, stiffness and joint changes, loin coldness, hernias, testicular problems, libido weakness, and urogenital symptoms in general.

General Symptoms

Low blood pressure, nonpsychosomatic asthma, vomiting, and chest pain.

Coupled minor chakra	Clavicular
Coupled major chakra	Brow
Meridian	Liver
Acupoint location	ST 30 (symphysis pubis)
Key point	PC 7
Time of maximum energy	2:00–4:00 a.m.
Color	Indigo
Sound pitch	A
Vibrational rate (radionics)	228893
Homeopathic remedy	*Juniperus comm.*

Clavicular Chakra

The Clavicular chakra is situated at the medial end of the clavicle at point KID 27. It is associated with the Groin and Brow chakras (see Figure 2.14).

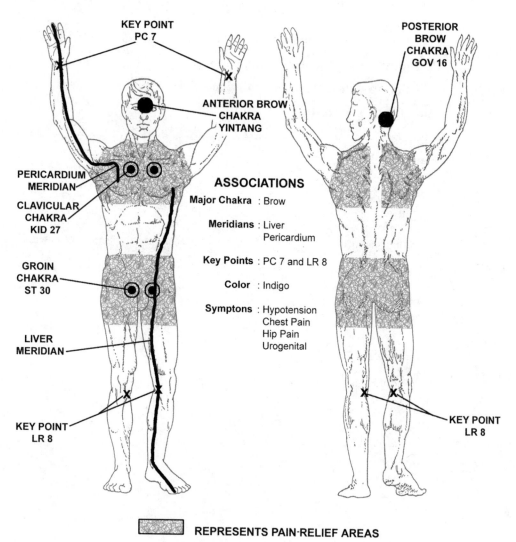

REPRESENTS PAIN-RELIEF AREAS

FIGURE 2.14

Associations of the Groin and Clavicular Chakras

Local Symptoms

Chest pains, thyroid imbalance, lower cervical stiffness, sternal pain, and sternoclavicular joint pain.

General Symptoms

The symptoms are the same as those listed under Groin chakra, with the addition of generalized bony abnormalities due to the imbalance of calcium metabolism, for example; Scheuermann's disease; and ankylosing spondylitis.

Coupled minor chakra	Groin
Coupled major chakra	Brow
Meridian	Pericardium
Acupoint location	KID 27 (medial aspect of clavicle)
Key point	LR 8
Time of maximum energy	4:00–6:00 a.m.
Color	Indigo
Sound pitch	A
Vibrational rate in radionics	116845
Homeopathic remedy	*Cimicifuga racemosa*

Shoulder Chakra

The Shoulder chakra is a very powerful chakra situated at the tip of the shoulder at point LI 15. It is associated with the Navel and Throat chakras. (See Figure 2.15.)

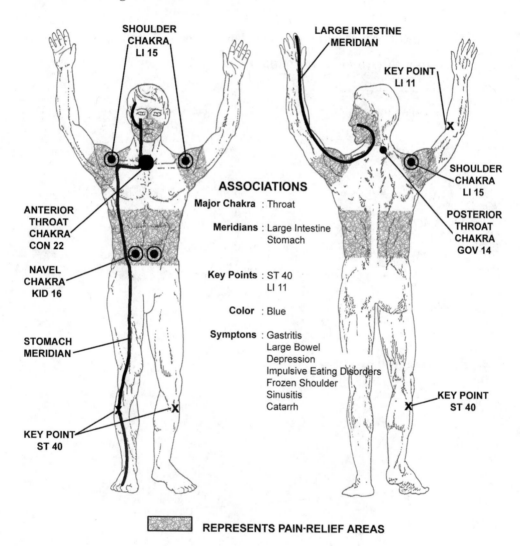

FIGURE 2.15

Associations of the Shoulder and Navel Chakras

Local Symptoms

Pain in the shoulder joint, with or without joint changes and stiffness, and frozen shoulder.

General Symptoms

Gastritis, small and large bowel symptoms and pain, constipation, chronic diarrhea, diverticulitis, deep depression, eating disorders.

Coupled minor chakra	Navel
Coupled major chakra	Throat
Meridian	Large Intestine
Acupoint location	LI 15 (tip of shoulder)
Key point	ST 40
Time of maximum energy	6:00–8:00 a.m.
Color	Blue
Sound pitch	G
Vibrational rate (radionics)	888735
Homeopathic remedy	*Platina*

Navel Chakra

The Navel chakra is situated just by the navel (umbilicus) at point KID 16. It is associated with the Shoulder and Throat chakras (see Figure 2.15).

Local Symptoms

Localized pain around the umbilicus, irritable bowel syndrome, and ileocaecal valve syndrome.

General Symptoms

These symptoms are the same as those listed under Shoulder chakra, with the addition of general weariness and some symptoms associated with anorexia.

Coupled minor chakra	Shoulder
Coupled major chakra	Throat
Meridian	Stomach
Acupoint location	KID 16 (by the navel)
Key point	LI 11
Time of maximum energy	8:00–10:00 a.m.
Color	Blue
Sound pitch	G
Vibrational rate (radionics)	114969
Homeopathic remedy	*Plumbum*

Ear Chakra

The Ear chakra is situated just behind the earlobe at the powerful point of TE 17. It is associated with the Heart and Intercostal chakras. (See Figure 2.16.)

Local Symptoms

Localized ear swellings, mastoiditis, torticolis, tinnitus, mild deafness of a traumatic etiology, otitis media, Bell's palsy, dizziness, and light-headedness.

General Symptoms

Eye strain, cataract, thoracic pain, stiffness and joint changes, lower rib pain, diaphragmatic pain and stitch, and head shingles.

Coupled minor chakra	Intercostal
Coupled major chakra	Heart
Meridian	Gallbladder
Acupoint location	TE17 (behind ear)
Key point	TE 4
Time of maximum energy	10:00 p.m.–12:00 a.m.
Color	Green
Sound pitch	F
Vibrational rate (radionics)	665689
Homeopathic remedy	*Baryta Carb.*

Intercostal Chakra

The Intercostal chakra is situated in the midaxillary line in the sixth intercostal space at point SP 21. It is associated with the Ear and Heart chakras. (See Figure 2.16.)

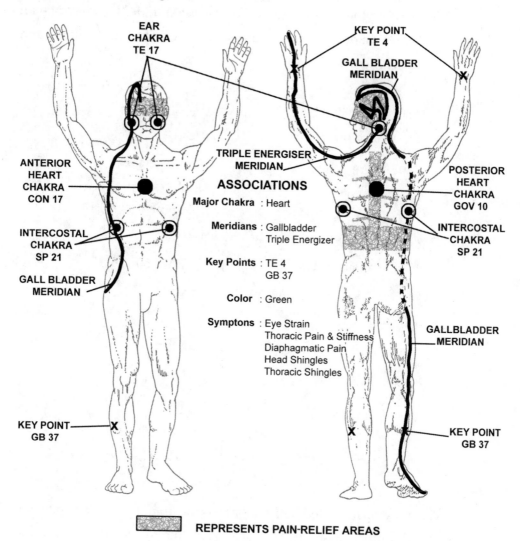

FIGURE 2.16

Associations of the Ear and Intercostal Chakras

Local Symptoms

Pain and discomfort in the chest, intercostal shingles.

General Symptoms

These symptoms are the same as those listed under Ear chakra, with the addition of general weakness and discomfort in the limbs and some febrile diseases.

Coupled minor chakra	Ear
Coupled major chakra	Heart
Meridian	Triple Energizer
Acupoint location	SP 21 (sixth intercostal space—midline)
Key point	GB 37
Time of maximum energy	12:00–2:00 a.m.
Color	Green
Sound pitch	F
Vibrational rate (radionics)	444661
Homeopathic remedy	*Kali carb.*

COMBINING MAJOR AND MINOR CHAKRAS

As previously stated, the minor chakras do not provide a gateway to the emotional body. However, each allows a penetration to the subtler edge of the etheric body, which makes them more powerful than the ordinary acupoints that are used for sedation and pain relief, or indeed the eight points that comprise the Key points of the extraordinary meridians. To review, where the minor chakras are given an association with a major chakra, this means that they represent reflected points of the majors; for example, the Hand and the Foot chakras at points PC 8 and KID 1 are the reflexes of the Crown at Gov 20, and so on. These force centers can easily be combined into treatment formulae to provide six very powerful modalities that can be used in physical therapy and acupuncture when treating most conditions that you encounter. When combinations of the chakras are used, the treatment of more chronic diseases is possible. To refresh your memory, here are the combinations once again:

- The Spleen minor chakra is associated with Sacral/Solar Plexus major chakras.
- The Hand/Foot minor chakras are associated with Crown major chakra.
- The Elbow/Knee minor chakras are associated with Base major chakra.
- The Groin/Clavicular minor chakras are associated with Brow major chakra.
- The Shoulder/Navel minor chakras are associated with Throat major chakra
- The Ear/Intercostal minor chakras are associated with Heart major chakra.

Symptoms of the Combined Chakras

The following sections represent just a few conditions that are treatable with combination chakra therapy. Details of the principles and practicalities of treatment will be given in the next chapter.

Crown/Hand/Foot

Head shingles, cervical spondylosis, metatarsalgia and other chronic foot maladies, vertigo, hypertension, chronic headaches, delusions, and symptoms related to some upper-motor neuron disease.

Brow/Clavicular/Groin

All chronic respiratory disease, all chronic throat conditions, migraines, catarrh, general infections and infectious diseases, altered hearing, dizziness, some chronic genitourinary conditions, and chronic low back pain.

Throat/Shoulder/Navel

Asthma, introversion, colitis and irritable bowel syndrome, diverticulitis, frozen shoulder, sinusitis, and paranoia.

Heart/Ear/Intercostal

Thoracic herpes, some facial neuralgia, general chronic heart and circulatory maladies, palpitation, varicosities, benign tumors and growths, and cysts.

Solar Plexus/Sacral/Spleen

Conditions of the autoimmune system, glandular fever, chronic fatigue syndrome, depression and worry, eczema, hay fever, lymphatic obstructions, menopausal and menstrual imbalances, impotence, symptoms of rheumatoid arthritis, edema, and water retention.

Base/Elbow/Knee

Chronic spinal conditions, ankylosing spondylitis, lumbar spinal arthritis and chronic low back pain, elbow and knee arthritis, lethargy, chronic cystitis, nephritis, depression, bone-related conditions, fractures (especially idiopathic and healing bone at a faster rate), and delusion.

Now that we have explored general chakra theory, in the following chapters we will take a look at the practical applications of these powerful centers and how they may be used in many of the hands-on healing modalities. As stated, the chakras may be used in many different healing modes, ranging from the hands-on to the hands-off treatments. I have put the practical chapters in the most natural order, starting with Chapter 3, "Bodywork and Acupressure," progressing through Chapter 4, "Reflexology," and ending with Chapter 5, "Healing" (which in turn is subdivided into sections on contact and noncontact techniques). I will also include some craniosacral philosophy, since it plays an integral part in the assessment and treatment methods.

As we know, the word *heal* means "to make whole"; therefore *all* of the modalities mentioned can be used in healing. I have used the word *healing* in the title of the final chapter to address the needs of countless numbers of practitioners who treat the energy body (physical and aura) with their hands. In no way do I mean to suggest that one modality of healing is superior to another. Each modality of using the chakra energy system is aimed at the therapist who feels most comfortable in practicing a particular type of therapy.

In this book I describe ways in which the chakras may be treated just by using the hands. Although each chapter describes a particular therapy, please do not assume that each should be used in isolation. There is no reason why combinations of the therapies described cannot be used within one treatment session. For example, in the treatment of, say, lower back pain, the practitioner can use bodywork chakra therapy, acupressure, reflexology, and healing to ease the symptoms and prevent further imbalance. In most chapters, I offer some case histories that pertain to each modality. Although I link certain conditions with each approach, this is purely for ease of understanding; it is not to say that other modalities would not be pertinent. Therefore, Chapter 3 naturally deals with mechanical and structural (musculoskeletal) conditions plus pain relief; chapter 4 covers both physical and emotional conditions, and Chapter 5 will deal mostly with emotional conditions and stress release. However, in each chapter it will be pointed out that no actual division exists between physical and emotional conditions—one may cause the other.

CHAPTER THREE

Bodywork and Acupressure

I have always thought myself fortunate that my original qualification in medicine was that of a chartered physiotherapist. While solely working in that specialization and since branching out into the fuller modality of natural medicine, I have always pioneered the use of the hands, having addressed countless conferences, courses, and workshops where the use of touch has been stressed. On numerous occasions I have implored physical therapists to throw away their electrical gadgetry and just to concentrate on using their hands as a genuine effective healing modality.

I am just one of very many physical therapists worldwide to have spread his wings into the study and practice of acupuncture. Many newly qualified acupuncturists seem to be obsessed with needles. Traditional Chinese Medicine, however, is a broad-spectrum healing modality consisting of needles, moxa, herbs, diet, *and* pressure. Many ancient pressure techniques have been handed down through the ages to become individual therapies in their own right. These include meridian acupressure, reflexology, tsubo point pressure, Tui Na, shiatsu, Indian head massage, and the newer ones based on "touch for health" and applied kinesiology. All these pressure and massage techniques have a place, and each is effective in the correct hands (no pun intended).

Touch therapy and massage are great modalities in their own right, but with the added dimension of working with the body's subtle energy system, the results obtained through these therapies can be considerably enhanced. The word *acupressure* often seems inadequate in describing this approach. It is, in fact, a total all-encompassing system of medicine. In this chapter we will discuss the treatment of musculoskeletal and pain conditions using body-work acupressure with the chakra energy system. I am not inferring that musculoskeletal conditions can be treated only through the use of these methods, nor that other types of illnesses cannot be treated with acupressure.

BODYWORK

Many different styles of bodywork can be used with the chakra energy system. The main ones are massage (in various forms), the mobilizing of joints and vertebrae, applied kinesiology, polarity therapy, and gentle manipulation or adjustments. Osteopaths and chiropractors reading this book will already know the history of the two main manipulation disciplines. Some physical therapists and other body workers, however, may not realize that their origins are grounded in energy medicine and holism. D. D. Palmer is generally credited with having founded chiropractic. In 1895 he adjusted the third cervical vertebra of a deaf janitor, thereby restoring his hearing. Palmer insisted that there was a vital force or energy called *innate*. The innate was the power that kept the autonomic system functioning and expressed itself through the nervous system. He stated that chiropractic in itself does not cure; the adjustment relieves and removes the cause, then the life force, or innate, transmits impulses without hindrances and effects a cure. Of course, many modern types and philosophies of chiropractic do not adhere to the "energy" body concept.

Andrew Taylor Still was the founder of osteopathy. He went to medical school and then into the army, where he rose to the rank of major and became an army surgeon. He came to believe that a person should be treated as a whole, that patients cannot get sick in one area of the body without the involvement of other parts. Still developed the art of manipulative therapy based on his detailed knowledge of human anatomy, physiology, and the newly found interrelationship between the body and its function. He found that by carefully palpating a patient's soft tissues, he could ascertain organic imbalance and that by gently manipulating visceral and soft tissue, he could achieve startling results. Still lived to be eighty-nine years old and left a legacy of over eleven thousand osteopathic practitioners in the United States and Europe. He is still remembered today for his simple yet far-reaching statement: *Structure governs function.*

ACUPRESSURE

Acupressure has been used in healing for over five thousand years and has been a useful adjunct of therapy. Many types and ways of giving acupressure exist. This chapter will deal with the use of gentle touch and stimulation of the acupoints in balancing the body's energies. As we know, the main energy channels that house the vital force or chi are called meridians. There are fourteen named meridians, of which twelve are associated with organs that are understood in conventional medicine and two that are unilateral. There are also an additional six meridians that are mixes and composites of the others, making twenty meridians in all (eighteen bilateral, and two unilateral).

Acupoints (or *tsubo*) are located along the meridian channels in particular places on the skin. These are usually quite easy to find and detect in that they lie either proximal or distal to certain bony prominences or in hollows made naturally by muscular or tendinous intersections. The acupoints may be likened to the lock gates on a canal that allows water to flow through when activated, hence allowing energy to flow along the meridian. This, though, is a very simplistic way of looking at the subtle anatomy, especially when many scientists don't even believe that meridians even exist! Acupoints are tiny (approximately 1 millimeter in circumference) "fibrous" nodules that appear to have an internal energy connection with specific organs. My view regarding acupoints is that they are reflected points of the central and autonomic nervous system, hence working through the thalamus and the spinal cord. It is via the spinal connections that a "balance" of energy may occur. This is not to say that when acupoints are stimulated or held that the inner and outer economy at organic and auric levels are not also affected. It is a complicated area that future books, *The Chakra Energy System and Acupuncture* and *The Holistic Spine*, will cover in much more detail.

In balancing and treating, a therapist normally uses gentle touch when working with the chakras. The exception to this is when the Base chakra and other major chakra points need to be stimulated because of chronic conditions. When any major or minor chakra seems to be congested and in a "yin" state, the point needs to be stimulated in order to "create" a reservoir of energy.

Feel

With very few exceptions, acupressure is *not* simply a watered-down version of acupuncture. I have shouted this from the rooftops for the past thirty odd years. One exception would be the treatment of chronic neurological conditions or where using a needle is the best option, because of the point's location (e.g., the use of Bladder 1 (which is located in the inner canthus of the eye). When you are using acupressure and energy bodywork of any type, you will gain a real *feel* for the energies that you are attempting to affect. In acupuncture, the only true guideline as to whether the energy flow has been affected is by the "take" on the needle or the "te-chi" sensation. This takes time to practice and is a difficult sensation to ascertain in every point on the body. Although acupuncture is a very effective modality in balancing and treating the chakra energy system, there is no doubt that acupressure and the "hands-on" approach is superior in many ways.

It is vital that the therapist has a "feel" for the patient and that the patient has a "feel" for the therapist. It's a two-way thing. As stated before, with acupressure, one can actually *feel* the energies and *knows* when an energy balance has taken place and where there is harmony. The sensation of feel can be interpreted in many different ways. The following are the most common sensations when the fingers or hands are placed on the skin:

1. A slight pulsing underneath the fingers will eventually become a balanced pulsing under both fingers; that is, the pulsing may start off being irregular but becomes even after a while. When the pulses are equal in strength, a harmony or energy balance exists between the two points, and you may feel a "oneness" of both fingers/hands.

2. With or without pulsing, a sensation of heat, which often has a slow buildup, may also be experienced. Skeptics would say that this represents the conduction heat of body contact (and, of course, they would be correct), but in reality it is much more than that.

The sensation becomes harmonious. When the heat surges and the pulsings are equal, you *know* that an energy balance has occurred. The *change of emphasis* (described in the next section) often occurs. Although it is quite permissible for you to move on to the next stage of the treatment shortly after an energy balance has been achieved, it is not a bad idea to keep contact for a few more seconds. Doing so results in a harmonious sensation for the patient and provides a feeling of relaxation and well-being. Your hands or fingers will often seem as if they are glued to the patient's skin.

3. You may also experience a sensation along the course of a meridian line or other invisible energy lines. This could be like "water trickling" or "electric shock" or just simply a pleasant and harmonious glow. It is very important to be in contact with the correct acupoint when performing acupressure. The results will not be as strong if your finger is slightly out. As with acupuncture, although there is an area of influence around each acupoint, obviously it is always best to be spot-on.

The patient also receives certain signals that the treatment is working. He or she may feel heat under your fingers or a "trickling" of energy flow from one finger to the other. A patient who is used to this type of treatment will know instinctively when an energy balance has been achieved and will often say so. All massage and hands-on techniques come with experience—performing acupressure using the chakra energy system is no exception to this.

Change of Emphasis

The term *change of emphasis* describes the change that takes place within the brainwave frequency of both the patient and the therapist. Each person (and animal) experiences different levels of consciousness that correspond with their brainwave frequency and breathing pattern at the time. Table 3.1 below explores these different levels of consciousness.

TABLE 3.1. LEVELS OF CONSCIOUSNESS

State of Consciousness	Brainwave Frequency	Breathing Rhythm	State of Being
Active thinking	Beta 13 to 30 cycles per second (cps)	Inhale 1 to 2 seconds Exhale 1 to 2 seconds	Questioning, thinking
Predrowsy	Alpha 8 to 13 cps	Inhale 8 seconds Exhale 8 seconds	Daydreaming
Change of emphasis "healing"	Alpha/Theta 7.8 cps	Inhale 4 seconds Exhale 8 seconds	Transition from personal to transpersonal
Drowsy	Theta 4 to 8 cps	Inhale 4 seconds Exhale 16 seconds	Transpersonal, creative, intuitive
Sleep	Delta 0.5 to 4 cps	Inhale 4 seconds Exhale up to 30 seconds	Restful body and mind, harmony, peace

Let us analyze the above table. Our normal everyday level of consciousness, in which we breathe, think, and have our being, is Beta state. Our brainwave activity in this state is between thirteen and thirty cycles per second (cps). (Cps is often referred to as hertz). In cases of hyperactivity and anxiety, the top figure may reach over ninety cps, although this is rare. Many times during our working day, we may drift slightly out of structured conscious thought. This is called the Alpha state, which resonates at between eight and thirteen cps. The breathing pattern in this state also becomes much longer, in in- and out-breaths. We move into Alpha state more times in the day than we realize—this state may last a split second, or it could last for several minutes. It often occurs when we are doing something routine and "boring." An example of this would be traveling along a familiar stretch of road and suddenly becoming aware that we have covered the previous half-mile without any conscious awareness of doing so. Staying in this kind of prolonged Alpha state could have dire consequences!

As discussed earlier, the next state of consciousness is called the Alpha/Theta (A/T) state. A patient may experience this state during any natural medicine therapy treatment in which the emphasis is on producing relaxation and healing. The A/T state may therefore occur during acupressure, reflextherapy, healing, and acupuncture. It is in these first three touch therapies that the change may be felt by both the therapist and the patient simultaneously. Only the patient feels the A/T state in acupuncture. In touch therapy, when your fingers or hands are in contact with the patient for any length of time (at least two minutes), you "tune in" to the patient's energy flow, either that of the whole body or that of the specific system that is being addressed. A harmony is produced between you and the patient when both of you have a brain wave frequency of 7.8 cps (A/T state). *True healing and oneness cannot take place until this state of harmony is achieved!*

At this frequency, both therapist and patient are in a state of relaxation. In practical acupressure, reflexology, and contact healing, the sensation experienced is quite marked (even taking into account the subtlety of what is occurring). A "shift" of sensation seems to take place under the fingers or hand—with lovely gentle warmth where there was none before. The tissues seem to change their texture and become like warm "putty," with your fingers able to "sink in" to the tissues a little more. Often, though not always, the patient too will feel this change. The A/T state heralds the time of oneness between the therapist and the patient.

The phrase "change of emphasis" or "shift of emphasis" will be used several times in this book, and it is essential that you learn to feel the difference between this state and the "normal" energy balancing occurring in acupressure and reflexology where there is "just" a similarity of sensation under the fingers. If you place your fingers or hands on the acupoints or reflexes for too long following the A/T state, the patient may very well nod off. This is an encouraging sign when it occurs. It shows that he or she is very relaxed and has the utmost confidence in you, the practitioner. The next state of consciousness is the Theta state, which resonates at four to eight cps. This is a presleep and very drowsy state. This is also the state in which meditation takes place, although some very experienced meditators may attain this state during any level of consciousness. Often, though in the Theta state, the person feels very light and sometimes detached from the physical plane of being. Some people have had out-of-body experiences while in this state. The final state of consciousness is Delta, which resonates at between 0.5 and 4 cps. Exhalations are very long in this state—which is another way to say sleep.

Rules

There are some golden rules that should be observed, which will make for better and speedier treatments:

1. Do not try too hard by "willing" the energy flow and balance to occur and the patient to improve. Concentration is all-important,

but with time, the healing energy will flow and the points will balance, so do not rush it.

2. Keep your mind on the patient—do not let it wander. This does not mean that you should maintain blind concentration to the abandonment of all else, but focusing on the job at hand does seem to achieve better results.

3. Use the same fingers in balancing, for example, either the index fingers of both hands or the middle fingers of both hands. If you use odd fingers, an energy balance will not be achieved as quickly. This is because there is a negative or positive magnetic polarity to each finger. Energy flows from negative to positive—the left index finger has a positive polarity, and the right index finger has a negative polarity, so by using the same fingers, a better energy balance may be achieved. I prefer to use the middle fingers in most treatment scenarios. Do what feels most comfortable.

4. With most acupressure techniques used with the chakras, employ a *very* light touch. Remember that *subtle* energy is being manipulated! Do not "skin polish" or massage holes into the patient's skin. The very lightest of touches with the finger pad is all that will be required while balancing. During the opening phases of treating chronic conditions, this technique changes—more on that later. I have had to scold many of my students, who are physical therapists or osteopaths, for their lack of *feel* for skin textures. These practitioners are indoctrinated in giving heavy manual body massage or tendinous frictions with no subtlety of approach. When these students learn the subtle approach, they are sometimes quite shocked to discover that it actually works. The therapist soon finds out that *subtle* means *power*, which means *results!*

Techniques

The same rules apply to using acupressure with the chakras as they do to using acupressure with the meridians. A thorough list of types and techniques appears in my first two books on acupressure and reflexology. The three main techniques that are used with the chakras are stimulation, sedation, and energy balancing. Let's take a look at them now.

1. *Stimulation.* Stimulation is usually performed with the finger pad of the forefinger or middle finger (sometimes the thumb). It consists of applying a constant uniform pressure on a single point, which is designed to "energize" the point. An example of this would be the stimulation of the posterior aspect of the Base chakra at the sacrococcygeal junction in order to put some energy into that point and subsequently into the chakra. This is one of the most common techniques used, especially with chronic conditions. It will be described in more detail later in this chapter.

2. *Sedation.* Sedation is performed by placing the tip of the middle finger or the whole palm placed over the physical chakra. It is done when there is too much energy either in the chakra or in the acupoint that is being treated. Hold the finger or hand on or over the point to be affected until you feel a difference of sensation. This can range from an increase of heat to a complete change of emphasis.

3. *Energy balancing.* Energy balancing is performed between two points, using either the finger pads or the whole hand. You will know when an energy balance has occurred when the sensations that are felt under each finger or hand is the same. This may take quite some time. It is important that you not will or encourage

this energy balance to occur in any way. The points will balance when they are good and ready. There are two aspects to be considered in energy balancing. First, a simple energy balance occurs fairly quickly (approximately one minute following contact). In most instances this is all that needs to happen before proceeding to the next stage of the treatment. The second aspect of energy balancing involves continually holding the points with your fingers or hands through the *change of emphasis,* the point of oneness between the therapist and patient when healing can begin to take place. This hold can take five minutes or more and often forms the backbone of the treatment of an individual chakra that is being balanced anteriorally and posteriorally.

So what can be achieved by using acupressure and bodywork with the chakra energy system? As was explained in the theory chapters, you are addressing the very *cause* of the energy imbalance, so using these types of therapy directly with the chakras can yield results that are unbelievable to some.

The remainder of the chapter will deal with practicalities of muscle energy balancing and stimulation; leg-length differentials; acute and chronic peripheral joint conditions; acute and chronic spinal conditions; and pain relief using the minor chakras and case histories.

MUSCLE ENERGY BALANCING AND MUSCLE STIMULATION

In this section we will look at the many aspects of treating muscle conditions using the chakra energy system.

Organic, Chakra, and Meridian Associations

Physical therapists used to be taught that muscular spasms around a lesion occurred as part of a self-healing mechanism of protection. They were taught to massage the spasm in order to "soften up" the muscle, hence allowing adequate flow of blood, lymph, and chi to the muscle and the underlying soft tissues, which would allow them to adjust joints that have been pulled out of alignment by the spasm. This was the cornerstone of the treatment of muscular imbalance by physical therapists, osteopaths, and chiropractors until the early 1960s. Although it often worked, the thrust of the treatment was very symptom oriented. Because the *cause* of the spasm had not been addressed, the underlying structures were still vulnerable to misalignments and possible subluxations. It also represented a very "Newtonian" way of *doing* something to the patient in sometimes quite a forceful manner in the "no pain, no gain" school.

It was in the early 1960s that Dr. George Goodheart came up with a new idea for working with muscles. Goodheart concluded that it wasn't really muscle spasm that caused pain and joint misalignments, but that weak muscles on one side of the body caused normal opposing muscles (antagonists) to become or seem tight. But when a muscle is tight or knotted, this indicates that the muscle is *weak*, not strong! Goodheart's research showed that most muscles have an energy association with internal organs via the meridian or "internal" energetic system. He devised the system of therapy called applied kinesiology (AK), an offshoot of modern chiropractic. According to AK, muscles may be "tested" to see how weak or strong they are, and it is the weak muscles that need to be "strengthened" in order to create a balance of energy in the muscle, organ, and meridian. This is not meant to be the type of muscle strength testing that physical therapists usually carry out, since it is certainly not a question of brute force; rather, it is a method of using very subtle holding techniques to ascertain if the muscle spindle contracts or "takes."

The association of each organ, meridian, and muscle is shown in Table 3.2. This table in no way covers every muscle in the body, but you should be able to use this knowledge in the treatment of 99 percent of all musculoskeletal conditions. This knowledge has profound implications in the treatment of these conditions. Many conditions that seem to be of a mechanical nature may *not* have a mechanical etiology. Rather, they may be caused by organic, chi, lymphatic, or emotional factors, and the seemingly mechanical condition is merely that the patient is housing the symptoms. It is therefore not always in his or her best interest to merely treat the symptoms without addressing the cause. A good way of ascertaining whether or not the cause is truly mechanical is to ask the patient how the condition occurred. If he or she replies that it was a direct injury, sprain, blow, or trauma, then you may treat the local symptoms by using any physical therapy method that has been tried-and true over the years. If, however, the reply is that "it just happened" or "it crept up slowly," then this indicates a non mechanical etiology, and the true cause needs to be addressed. Only by using the chakra energy system can this be done. Of course, the local symptoms have to be eased in order to help the patient, but unless the cause is located and the energy balanced, the symptoms will return.

Table 3.2 represents my own research over several years, based on the work of David Walther and John Thie et al. You will see that each vertebral level is associated with one or more muscle. This is where you use touch to create an energy balance within the muscle involved, the exact point of contact being the space below the spinous process of the vertebra. This point may also be used to analyze or "therapy localize." Please do not confuse the associated vertebra with the many nerve connections to a muscle originating in the spine—attempting to rationalize any neural connection will only confuse! Second, each muscle has an associated major and minor chakra that may be used in its strengthening and balancing. The physical representations of the chakras are used here, since they represent powerful acupoints that may be used to treat the cause of the problem. Previous research has shown the correlation between the muscles and meridians. You will note from Table 3.2 that each muscle has a different "formula" of relationships, thus making each muscular balance unique to that muscle. In contrast to methods used in traditional acupressure, there is no need to distinguish between sedation and stimulation of the energy flow to that muscle. By using the technique described below, you can balance the muscle energy—where it was once weak before, it becomes strong, and while it once was in spasm, it now becomes normal.

Treatment Method

1. Identify the muscle to be balanced. The muscle might need balancing because of pain, spasm, congestion, or because analysis has proven it to be weak. All muscles that have been subject to trauma are in a state of imbalance; this is particularly true after surgery. Treatment using this method saves hours if not days of muscle strengthening. It is hopeless in the extreme to try to strengthen a muscle by conventional means if there is an underlying trauma or

TABLE 3.2. CORRESPONDENCES OF MUSCLES, ORGANS, MERIDIANS, VERTEBRAE, AND MAJOR AND MINOR CHAKRAS

Muscle	Organ	Meridian	Vertebra	Major chakra	Minor chakra
Sternomastoid	Sinus	Stomach	C1	Crown	Ear
Facial	Sinus	Governor	C1-2	Crown	Ear
Neck, anterior and posterior	Sinus	Stomach	C1, 2, 3	Brow	Clavicular
Upper trapezius	Eye and ear	Kidney	C3	Crown	Ear
Supraspinatus	Brain	Conception	C4	Crown	Ear
Levator scapula	Parathyroid	Stomach	C5	Throat	Clavicular
Pectoralis major (clavicular)	Stomach	Stomach	C6	Throat	Shoulder
Pectoralis major (sternal)	Liver	Liver	C6	Throat	Clavicular
Biceps	Stomach	Stomach	C6	Throat	Elbow
Serratus anterior	Lung	Lung	C6	Throat	Shoulder
Subscapularis	Heart	Heart	C6	Throat	Shoulder
Infraspinatus	Thymus	Triple Energizer	C6	Throat	Shoulder
Brachialis	Stomach	Stomach	C6	Throat	Elbow
Brachioradialis	Stomach	Stomach	C6	Throat	Hand
Wrist extensors	Stomach	Stomach	C6	Throat	Hand
Triceps	Pancreas	Spleen	C7	Throat	Elbow
Trapezius (mid and lower)	Spleen	Spleen	C7	Throat	Shoulder
Supinator	Stomach	Stomach	C7	Throat	Hand
Latissimus dorsi	Pancreas	Spleen	C7	Throat	Intercostal

Muscle	Organ	Meridian	Vertebra	Major chakra	Minor chakra
Wrist flexors	Stomach	Stomach	C7	Throat	Hand
Deltoid	Lung	Lung	T1	Throat	Shoulder
Teres major	Spine	Governor	T1	Throat	Elbow
Teres minor	Thyroid	Triple Energizer	T1	Throat	Elbow
Rhomboids	Liver	Liver	T2	Throat	Hand
Sacrospinalis	Bladder	Bladder	T2-L3	Heart	Intercostal
Abdominals	Small intestine	Small intestine	T4-T12	Solar Plexus	Navel
Quadriceps	Small intestine	Small intestine	L1-2	Solar Plexus	Groin
Iliopsoas	Kidney	Kidney	L2	Sacral	Groin
Sartorius	Adrenals	Triple Energizer	L3	Sacral	Knee
Gracilis	Adrenals	Triple Energizer	L3	Sacral	Foot
Tibialis anterior	Bladder	Bladder	L4	Sacral	Foot
Adductors	Circulation	Pericardium	L4-5	Sacral	Knee
Tensor fascia latae	Large intestine	Large intestine	L5	Sacral	Knee
Gluteus medius	Sexual	Pericardium	L5	Sacral	Groin
Gluteus maximus	Sexual	Pericardium	S1	Sacral	Knee
Hamstrings	Large intestine	Large intestine	S1	Sacral	Knee
Tibialis posterior	Adrenals	Bladder	S1	Sacral	Foot
Peroneus longus	Bladder	Bladder	S1	Sacral	Foot
Gastrocnemius and soleus	Adrenals	Triple Energizer	S2	Sacral	Foot
Popliteus	Gallbladder	Gallbladder	S3	Sacral	Knee

energy imbalance. The method as described paves the way for rehabilitation to be more worthwhile and less painful.

2. Then stroke the associated meridian in the direction of energy flow. This can be done by a very gentle broad sweep of the hand along the bilateral meridian. It can be done over clothing, if the patient desires.

3. Find the relevant vertebral level and hold it by the pad of the middle finger (remember to touch the space inferior to the spinous process of the associated vertebra). In the case of multiple vertebral levels, as with the abdominals and sacrospinalis, each level must be balanced in turn. You then place the middle finger pad of the other hand on the relevant major chakra point (frontal aspect), and an energy balance is achieved by obtaining a similar sensation under each finger. It is not so important to go through a change of emphasis, but the longer you maintain the hold, the more effective will be the outcome. It is advisable to hold for at least one to two minutes or longer if the muscle is chronically imbalanced.

4. Keep the finger on the spinal point, and place the other middle finger pad on the associated minor chakra point. Again, balance these two points for at least one minute.

5. Finally, you will need to balance the points of the major and minor chakra points with each other. This should take very little time.

When you retest the muscle you will find it to be strong. While this all sounds a bit incredible, *it works!* Try it for yourself. You are now in a position to carry out further treatment on the muscle or other associated parts. It is also very useful to complete the treatment session by placing one hand (or finger if suitable) on the belly of the affected muscle and to energy balance it with the major chakra. Doing so enhances the treatment and is much appreciated by the patient, since up to now that muscle has not been touched.

At first glance Table 3.2 may seem a little daunting. There are a few ways of making its contents easier to remember. First, it is imperative that you know your anatomy; otherwise you will be completely lost. The origins and insertions of each muscle *must* be known. Second, you will be notice that, with a few exceptions, the majority of the muscles have the Throat or Sacral chakra as a balancing point. Most of the upper-body muscles are associated with the Throat chakra, and the lower body muscles with the Sacral chakra. These two points are very easy to find, as are the relevant minor chakra correspondences.

LEG-LENGTH DIFFERENTIALS

Most patients with spinal and pelvic-related conditions need to have leg length checked prior to treatment. It is most important that legs be as close to the same length as possible. Almost every person has some degree of leg-length differential (due to pelvic hitching) of up to half an inch, with few or no obvious problems. It is also true that, with some patients, even a half-inch imbalance can produce a pelvic or even an atlas lesion.

Measure the leg-length differential with the patient lying completely flat, either prone or supine, and in as straight a postural line from head to toe as possible. Leg lengths are measured at the prominence of the tibial (medial) malleolus and *not* at the base of the heel. Most patients with a spinal condition will exhibit at least one of the six different types of leg-length imbalance. Types 1–3, as listed below, are very common; the others are less so. The following technique used to involve employing the key points of the eight extraordinary meridians, but since I have discovered the chakra energy system and its use with acupressure, only two points need be used—the Hand chakra at PC 8 and the Foot chakra at KID1. It has saved so much time and trouble, and I hope it will do the same for every practitioner who uses it. Hold the points by using the pads of the middle fingers with very gentle pressure until a similar pulsing is obtained. It may take anywhere from a few seconds to up to a minute. Do not attempt to go through a change of emphasis using this technique; it isn't necessary. The results are sometimes instant and remarkable. Let us now take a look at the different ways to treat the six types of leg-length imbalances.

Type 1—Sacral Condition

The patient is prone. Examination reveals a long leg and low buttock on the same side. When the knees are flexed, this remains the same.

Treatment: Balance the Foot and Hand chakra points on the short leg side.

Type 2—Sacral Condition with Atlas Involvement

The patient is prone. Examination reveals a long leg and low buttock on the same side. When the knees are flexed, the long leg becomes short.

Treatment: Balance the Foot and Hand chakra points on the long leg side.

Type 3—General Spinal Condition

The patient is prone. Examination reveals a long leg and a high buttock on the same side.

Treatment: Balance the Foot chakra of the long-leg side with the Hand chakra of the short-leg side. If this doesn't do the trick, this would indicate an upper spinal condition. Then you can simply balance the two Hand chakra points.

Type 4—Lower Back Pain

The patient is supine. Examination reveals a short leg and a high iliac crest on the same side.

Treatment: Balance the Foot chakra and the Hand chakra on the short-leg side.

Type 5—Lower Back Pain, with Sciatica

The patient is supine. Examination reveals a short leg and a high iliac crest on the same side, with the patient complaining of sciatica along some or all of the nerve.

Treatment: Balance the Foot chakra and the Hand chakra on the short-leg side (as with Type 4), but then balance the Knee chakra (middle of popliteal fossa at BL 40) and the Foot chakra of the affected side.

Type 6—Differentials That Cannot Be Adjusted

Differentials that cannot be addressed may be due to a long-standing rheumatoid condition, ankylosing spondylitis, or even gross osteoarthritic changes in the hips or knees. They could also, of course, indicate a permanently altered leg differential due to an old injury such as a fractured pelvis, femur, or tibia.

Treatment: This type of differential cannot be altered, except through the careful fitting of external or internal heel raises.

The above procedures may, at first glance, seem quite complicated, but in practice they are very simple to do. Check the differentials at each visit, as they can and do change. This is particularly true if the patient has not consulted you for some time and/or if he or she is employed in a sedentary occupation. If the pelvis is misaligned, what hope is there for alignment further up the spine? If the pelvis is equated with the foundation of the building, then it makes sense to have strong and balanced foundations—if not, the upper stories of the building (lumbar, thoracic, and cervical spine) will be affected.

MUSCLE LESIONS

In this section we will look at the treatment of chronic muscle lesions and imbalance due to scar tissue, fibrositic nodules, lymphatic congestion, or unresolved muscle tears. This type of lesion is usually very difficult to treat, and many treatment hours are often spent in deep massage and electrotherapy before the situation resolves itself. For information about the acupressure approach in other muscle lesions such as tendonitis and acute hematoma, please consult my first book, *Acupressure: Clinical Applications in Musculo-Skeletal Conditions.*

Principles of Treatment

1. To establish, as much as possible, a functional muscle.
2. To increase the blood and lymphatic circulation in the congested area.
3. To increase the chi flowing to the area and to make sure that the functional muscle aligns with other body structures.

Treatment Method

1. Both you and your patient should be comfortable. Massage the affected area with oil to improve the circulation and to start to ease congestion.

2. Locate the nearest chakra points either side of the muscle that is being treated and press these gently with the pads of the middle fingers until an energy balance is felt. The chakras can be major, minor, or a mix—it does not matter. An example of this would be to hold and balance the Knee and Foot chakra in the case of a torn gastrocnemius or soleus muscle, or to hold and balance the posterior Solar Plexus and Base chakras in the case of lumbar fibrositic nodules. There are many, many other possibilities, which cannot all be listed here.

3. When the energy balance has been attained and a definite constant pulsing felt underneath both fingers, slowly and methodically draw one of your fingers (usually on the dominant hand) supported by the adjacent fingers from one chakra to the other. There has to be a certain amount of depth to this, that is, the muscle needs to be affected, not just the skin. The fingers on the "doing" hand must have oil on them so as to make it easier for the patient— it will not impede what the practitioner feels, it will actually enhance it. While the same depth of contact is maintained and the dominant hand moves slowly toward the other hand, the pulsing under the fingers will be maintained. This is a sign that an adequate energy flow exists under the fingers.

   As the lesion appears under the dominant fingers (yes, it is possible to actually feel old muscle tears and deep scar tissue), you will find that the pulsing will stop. This indicates that the muscle tissue has changed in its texture and that this is the area that needs to be concentrated on. As soon as the pulsing stops under the "doing" finger, stop the movement. Wait for up to twenty seconds to reestablish the pulsing. This occurs in about 80 percent of cases. Where a pulsing does not materialize after twenty seconds or so, the distal fingers still on the other chakra point should be stimulated, along with the local fingers on the lesion. This may have to be done over a few ten second bursts of stimulation with the fingers before the pulsing resumes. This procedure needs to be repeated every time the pulsing disappears. Using this method you are totally in charge of the procedure; there is no hit or miss. The fingers do not lie!

Proceed with the "doing" hand until both hands close in on each other at the distal end. On a long deep scar or tear, the whole procedure may take several minutes. Round off the treatment by "energizing" the muscle concerned, as per the previous section.

If the technique is carried out correctly, you will usually need just one treatment session to completely restore full function to the affected muscle. Not only will the patient find that the affected muscle will be returned to normal, but also, because the muscle has been energy balanced with its correspondences, they will feel immeasurably better in themselves.

PERIPHERAL JOINT CONDITIONS

I have coined the treatment of joint conditions (spinal and peripheral) "Chinese physical therapy" or "Chinese osteopathy"—depending on the students at a particular workshop. I have come up with these terms because of the use of TCM philosophy in the field of bodywork. It may be appropriate to call the use of the chakras in the field of acupressure and bodywork "Indian physiotherapy," although that could be stretching things a little! Just to remind you of the main points used in peripheral joint conditions:

1. The Hand chakra—PC 8—is situated in the middle of the palm (stigmata point).
2. The Elbow chakra—PC 3—is situated in the middle of the cubital fossa just to the lateral aspect of the biceps tendon.
3. The Shoulder chakra—LI 15—is situated at the anterior and inferior border of the acromioclavicular joint, inferior to the acromion, when the arm is in abduction.
4. The Posterior Throat chakra—Gov 14—is situated between the spinous processes of the seventh cervical and first thoracic vertebrae in the midline.
5. The Posterior Sacral chakra—Gov 3—is situated between the spinous processes of the fourth and fifth lumbar vertebrae in the midline.
6. The Groin chakra—ST 30—is three finger widths (two cun) lateral to the upper aspect of the symphysis pubis.
7. The Knee chakra—BL 40—is situated in the middle of the popliteal fossa behind the knee.
8. The Foot chakra—KID 1—is situated on the sole of the foot in the midline, two thirds of the way up from the heel.

Principles of Treatment

1. To create a balance of energy (chi) through and in the affected joint to improve circulation of blood and lymph and to relieve congestion.
2. To reduce pain, swelling, and inflammation and to improve joint range and function in the affected joint.
3. To energy balance the improved joint with its coupled areas.

Order of Treatment

1. Massage the meridians that pass over and through the affected joint, in the direction of energy flow. (See Figure 3.1.)
2. Stimulate massage the distal chakra to create a reservoir of energy in the limb.
3. Balance energy *through* the affected joint between the distal chakra and the proximal chakra.
4. Balance energy between the painful point on the joint (lesion) and the distal chakra.
5. "Unwind" the affected joint in two aspects.
6. Balance the treated joint with its coupled reflexes.

Explanation of Treatment

1. Although the chakra energy system is a very powerful stand-alone tool for healing, the use of the meridians helps enhance the energy flow through the joint. The meridians do not have to be learnt exactly as they do in the study of acupuncture; you just need to understand the generalized flow that is needed. You may use your whole hand, and it can be performed over light clothes but is best done on the skin. It is most important that you perform the massage in the direction of the energy flow, as outlined in Figure 3.1, so as to maximize the chi flow within the joint. It is, obviously, an excellent idea to massage all fourteen (twelve bilateral and two unilateral) main meridians at the start of each treatment session, but this is usually impractical. It is vital, though, to massage the ones that pass over the affected joint, smoothly sweeping each meridian from first point to last point three or four times.

   On the arm the three yin meridians may be incorporated in one sweep of the hand from the shoulder and face toward the hand; likewise you may incorporate the three yang meridians with one sweep from the fingers toward the shoulder and face. The leg meridians are generally further apart and may require two or three sweeps on both yin and yang meridians. However

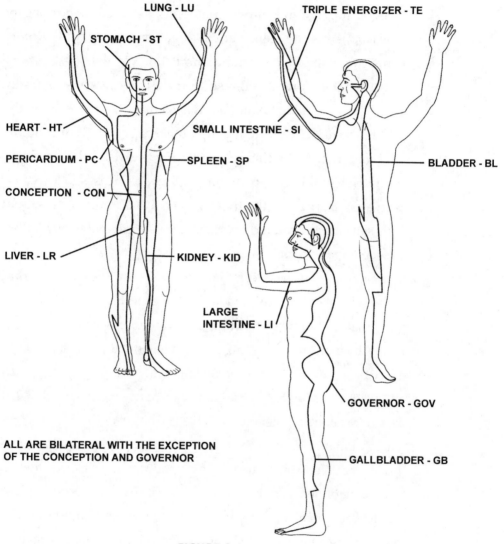

FIGURE 3.1
Traditional Chinese Meridian Channels

you decide to do it, the procedure does not take very long. This technique is useful both energetically and psychologically. It is a great way for you to "introduce yourself" to the patient and for him or her to initially receive "touch" therapy.

2. The next stage is to stimulate massage the distal chakra point. In all cases of subacute and chronic conditions, this needs to be done for at least one minute using simple finger-pad massage. The more chronic the condition, the more stimulation you will need to carry out. It is not important at this stage of the treatment to specifically place the "nondoing" hand, but it is comforting to hold it on the affected joint. It is essential that you get a feel for what is occurring underneath the finger stimulating the distal chakra. Some warmth should build up after a few seconds. This is followed by a greater elasticity of the tissues, even a "soft putty" sensation. This sensation of altered awareness must be experienced before proceeding to the next stage.

3. The next stage is to energy balance between the distal chakra (which has been stimulated and still has a finger on it) and the proximal chakra point through the joint. Energy balance the two points by using the same fingers of each hand. It is perfectly OK to place the whole hand over the chakra points or even to use a spread of two or three fingers instead of just one finger pad—just do what is comfortable and what feels right. The object of the exercise is to energy balance *through* the affected joint. This represents probably the hardest part of the whole procedure and is especially taxing for beginners to subtle bodywork. The overriding principle is to "let it happen" and not to force or to influence anything. The energy levels are bound to be sluggish in chronic joint imbalances, so energy is not going to flow quickly or easily.

Initially, there may be a great divergence of sensation between the fingers or hands—one may be pulsing warm, while the other may be pulsing cold, or one may not have any sensation at all, and the other one may feel vibrant. With experience you will be able to tell when the balance is complete. There has to be unanimity between the hands, with the same sensation felt under each finger. A definite harmony should be felt between one hand and the other. The patient will often feel certain sensations such as warmth, the trickling of water, or even electric shocks. At this stage of the procedure try not to analyze too much of what is occurring in the patient's tissues; just accept it. It helps if there is thought intention and focus on the affected joint during all the stages, but particularly with this one. Energy flow through the joint has to be "visualized." Also, it is helpful to get the patient on your side by asking him or her to concentrate on the procedure. It is most important that the energy balancing has occurred before you proceed to the next stage.

4. The fourth stage begins the involvement of the affected joint and is concerned with balancing energy between it and the distal chakra (where one finger is still situated). The finger is placed on the painful area of the joint (lesion), since this is usually the area of congestion where the symptoms are housed. As with most painful areas, you should take care not to press too hard—light pressure is sufficient. After a few seconds a similar sensation will be felt to the one achieved in stage 3. The "hold" will probably take about two to three minutes, which is less that for stage 3, but here you are capitalizing on the energy level that has been achieved so far and concentrating on where it is needed most—that is, on the chronic joint condition. It is useful to keep the fingers in place

for longer than is required merely to balance energy—the longer the fingers are held in place, the warmer and more pliable the tissues will become, and the more comfortable the whole area will feel. A change of emphasis should be felt during this stage, and it is at this point that the patient will start to feel his or her pain diminishing.

5. The stage of "unwinding" may sound the most complicated, but in practice is usually the easiest. In all traumas of joints and muscles the body has accepted a particular postural code that it is now being exhibited. It is well-known that when a joint is injured or when arthritic changes start to occur, many postural changes accompany this, in the joint, its immediate surroundings, and sometimes in the body as a whole. This occurs quite naturally as the body's attempt to protect itself from further damage or trauma. The joint's surrounding ligaments and muscles become tighter, adapting to the prime postural positioning according to the strength of the individual muscles. To regain homoeostasis in the joint and its environ, there must first be a regaining of the original postural coding so as to allow comfort in the area and to prevent further damage.

The approach of unwinding is well-known to practitioners of craniosacral therapy, zero balancing, polarity therapy, and Bowen technique (to name just a few). The hands are placed on opposite sides of the joint and held there for about half a minute. Warmth will then be felt, and the tension in the joint will slowly ease by the joint unwinding itself. This will be a unique sensation to those of you who have not met it before, and it may take some time to master this technique. The joint is attempting to return to normality in a subtle and yet powerful way. Unwinding will not occur

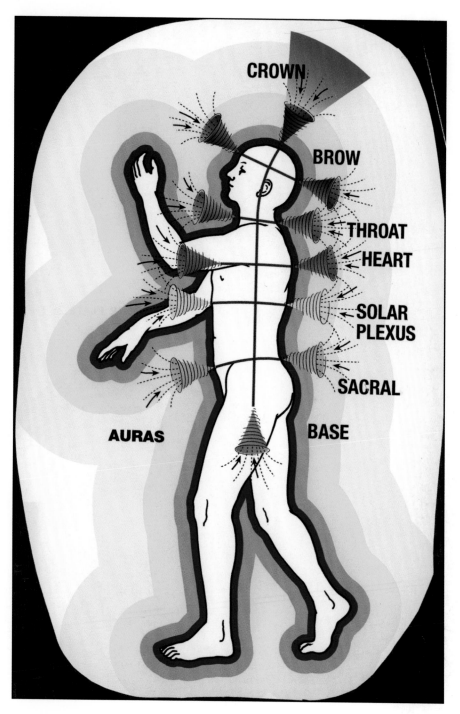

COLOR PLATE 1: *The Major Chakras and the Aura*

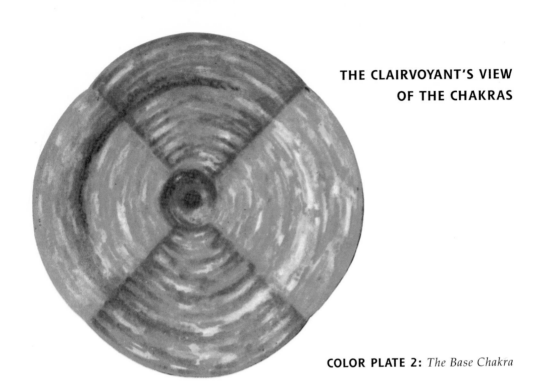

COLOR PLATE 2: *The Base Chakra*

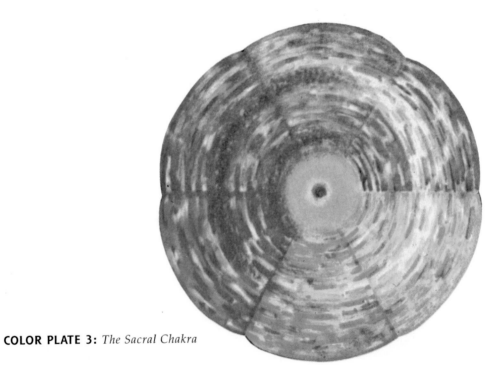

COLOR PLATE 3: *The Sacral Chakra*

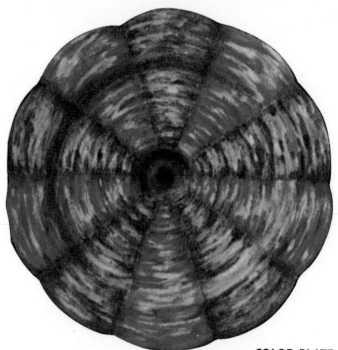

COLOR PLATE 4: *The Solar Plexus Chakra*

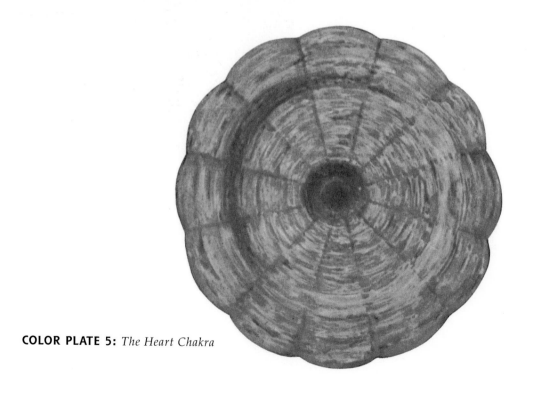

COLOR PLATE 5: *The Heart Chakra*

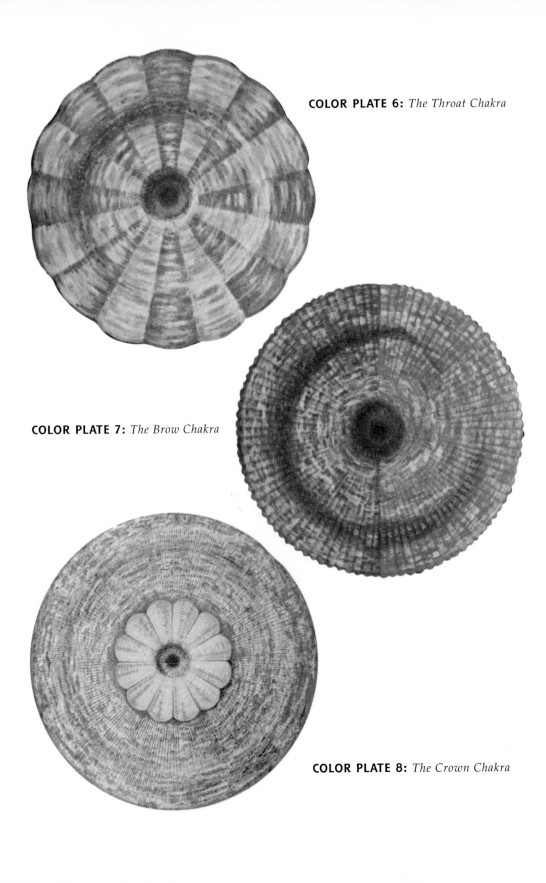

COLOR PLATE 6: *The Throat Chakra*

COLOR PLATE 7: *The Brow Chakra*

COLOR PLATE 8: *The Crown Chakra*

unless the previous stages have been completed—do *not* attempt to take shortcuts. Once again, my advice is to "let it happen" and not to attempt to move your hands against the natural movement of the joint. You are merely the instigator of this procedure that the patient is carrying out him- or herself—just sit back and let it happen. All you are doing is "changing a gear" in the patient's energy field to facilitate self-healing. The unwinding may take up to five minutes and will involve a change of hand positions until all four "corners" of the joint have been unwound. This whole concept of naturopathic healing may seem a little strange to some readers, especially to those of you who are used to "doing" things to your patient. Have no doubt, though, that energy medicine healing is the medicine of the future and will one day be accepted as standard procedure.

6. Following stages 1 to 5, the joint should now have more range of movement, less pain, and should generally feel more comfortable. Of course, it may take more than one treatment session to ease a joint that has been stiff and painful for many years. The joint now has to be energy balanced with its coupled joint, spinal chakra, and other associated reflexes (reflected areas). This procedure reinforces the previous work and enables the treated joint to become integrated with the rest of the body. It is important that this is done so as to give a much more balanced effect. The couples are (a) the parallel joint, (b) the opposite joint, (c) the associated spinal chakra, and (d) the appropriate reflexes. By parallel joint I mean that the upper limb joint is energy balanced with its couple on the leg and vice versa, for example, shoulder with hip, knee with elbow, wrist with ankle, and hand with foot. Opposite joint means just that—energy balance with the joint on the opposite side of the body, for

example, shoulder with shoulder, elbow with elbow, wrist with wrist, and hand with hand. The joint is then energy balanced with its associated spinal chakra. For the upper limb joints this is the posterior Throat chakra at C7-T1, and for the lower limb joints it is the posterior Sacral chakra at L4-5. These holds need just be done for about half a minute or so using the flat of the hand or the finger if the joint is too small for the whole hand to encompass it. The reflected point or pathway could be on the foot, hand, skull, leg, or arm. The most appropriate one will be mentioned in the next section dealing with treatment of specific joints.

SPECIFIC JOINT CONDITIONS
Shoulder Joint

Conditions that you may be called on to treat would include "frozen shoulder," osteoarthritis, supraspinatus and biceps tendonitis, and acromio-clavicular lesion. Although the last condition does not always involve the shoulder capsular ligament and is not strictly a shoulder lesion, the treatment theory is the same.

Order of Treatment

(See Figure 3.2.)

1. Massage the Large Intestine, Small Intestine, Gallbladder, Triple Energizer, Lung, Heart, and Pericardium meridians in the direction of the energy flow. Please note that in the case of very acute lesions, the meridian is massaged against the flow of energy in short strokes next to the joint.

2. Stimulate the Elbow chakra (PC3—situated in the center of the cubital fossa).

3. Energy balance between the Elbow chakra and the posterior Throat chakra at the cervicothoracic junction (Gov 14) through the lesion at the shoulder.

4. Energy balance between the shoulder lesion (at the "pain" point, or in the case of a chronic frozen shoulder, over the anterior aspect) and the Elbow chakra until a change of emphasis has been attained.

5. Unwind the shoulder joint, (a) with one hand placed over the lateral aspect of the shoulder (over the Shoulder chakra at LI 15) and the other placed over the posterior Throat chakra at the cervicothoracic junction (b) with the hands opposing each other placed on the anterior and posterior aspects of the joint.

6. (a) Energy balance with the hip joint on the same side of the body. (b) Energy balance with the opposite shoulder. (c) There is no need to energy balance with the posterior Throat chakra, since this has already been done. (d) Energy balance with the shoulder reflexes on the foot and lower leg.

Each energy balance should be held for no longer than thirty seconds until a similarity of sensation is felt under each hand. It is, though, important to hold the hand over the shoulder lesion and to place the other hand over the appropriate part of its reflex. In the case of anterior shoulder pain this would be energy balanced with the anterior aspect of the hip (Groin chakra) and anterior aspect of the other shoulder. If the lesion is on the lateral aspect (possible a/c joint lesion), this would be energy balanced with the lateral aspect of the hip and the same area of the other shoulder.

Elbow Joint

Conditions of the elbow would include Tennis elbow (lateral aspect inflammation), Golfer's elbow (medial aspect inflammation), and generalized capsulitis due to a repetitive strain syndrome. Be sure to ascertain whether the pain in the elbow is due to referred pain from the neck (as is the case with shoulder pain also). The treatment suggested should ease even referred pain temporarily, but the lower cervical spine should also be addressed.

Order of Treatment

(See Figure 3.2.)

1. Stroke the Heart, Pericardium, Lung, Triple Energizer, Large Intestine, and Small Intestine meridians in the direction of their energy flow. These need only be stroked between the fingers and the shoulder.

2. Stimulate the distal chakra point of PC 8 (Hand chakra, palm of hand).

3. Energy balance between the Hand chakra and the Shoulder chakra at LI 15 through the lesion at the elbow.

4. Energy balance between the Hand chakra and the "pain point" of the elbow until a change of emphasis is attained.

5. Unwind the joint. You can usually achieve this simply by placing the hands over the medial and lateral aspects of the joint.

6. (a) Energy balance with the respective part of the knee joint on the same side of the body. (b) Energy balance with the same aspect of the opposite elbow. (c) Energy balance with the posterior Throat chakra. This can be particularly effective if the pain is actually coming from this area of the neck, as with Golfer's elbow with a C7-T1 nerve root referral. (d) Energy balance with the elbow reflex on the foot and the leg. Experience has shown that these are the best reflexes to use.

Wrist Joint

Conditions to be considered here would be repetitive stress syndrome, other forms of tenosynovitis, carpal tunnel syndrome, and chronic edema of the wrist.

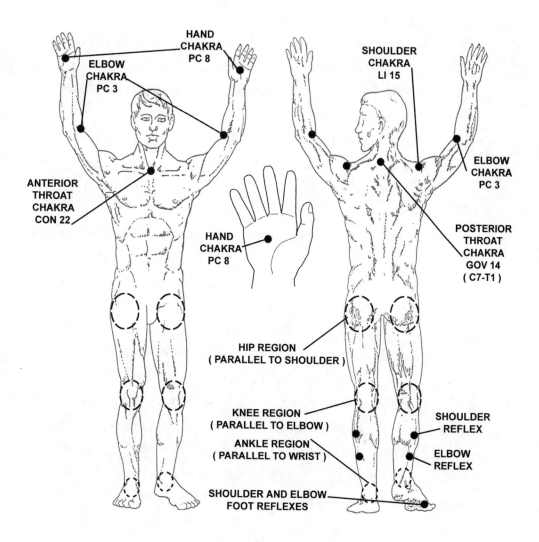

FIGURE 3.2

Points Used in the Treatment of Shoulder, Elbow, and Wrist Conditions

Order of Treatment

(See Figure 3. 2.)

1. Stroke the same meridians that were used in the elbow joint treatment in the direction of the energy flow. These need only be stroked between the fingers and the elbow.

2. Stimulate the Hand chakra at point PC 8 in the palm of the hand.

3. Energy balance between the Hand chakra and the Elbow chakra at PC 3 in the middle of the cubital fossa through the wrist lesion.

4. Energy balance between the pain point and the Hand chakra until a change of emphasis is reached. Please note that these two points could be adjacent (especially with carpal tunnel syndrome), and you should take care not to overlap the two.

5. Unwind the joint. This is only possible using the anterior and posterior aspects.

6. (a) Energy balance with the corresponding aspect of the ankle on the same side of the body. Please note that the anterior aspect of the wrist corresponds with the medial aspect of the ankle and that the posterior aspect of the wrist corresponds to the lateral aspect of the ankle. If you have any confusion over which aspect of the joint should be used to balance, remember that in all joint lesions, the reflex *will* be tender. This should make it much easier to find the point to use. (b) Energy balance with the same aspect of the opposite wrist joint. (c) Energy balance with the posterior aspect of the Throat chakra. (d) Energy balance with the wrist reflex on the lower part of the leg. In the case of carpal tunnel syndrome, the reflected area is the Achilles tendon.

Hip Joint

Pain in the hip may be caused by osteoarthritic changes in the joint itself, by pelvic congestion and inflammation to the sacroiliac and lumbosacral junction (referred pain), or by inflammation with mis-alignment of the femoral head as a result of a direct blow to the hip or of trauma to the knee or ankle. Because the hip joint is so deep within the pelvis it presents a formidable challenge to doing this type of work. With just a little patience, however, there can be great rewards for both you and your patient.

Order of Treatment

(See Figure 3.3.)

1. **Stroke** the Gallbladder, Stomach, and Bladder meridians in the direction of the energy flow. These meridians need to be stroked between the toes and the chest only. Pay particular attention to the Gallbladder meridian, the only one to pass through the hip joint.

2. **Stimulate** the Knee chakra at BL 40 (situated in the center of the popliteal fossa). Although the Knee chakra is the correct distal chakra point to use to create a reservoir of energy, it is usually advantageous to stimulate the posterior Base chakra (just above the coccyx) in all cases of chronic arthritis as well as the Knee. There are a few reasons for this. First, the Base chakra should be stimulated in all cases of chronic joint pain. Second, osteoarthritis in the hip is often associated with generalized pelvic congestion and tightness, and these will be relieved by stimulating the point. When you use the posterior Base chakra, the patient must be placed on his or her side lying for ease of access to the points. For the remainder of the treatment, use the Knee chakra as the distal chakra, since the Base chakra will be used later on in the treatment.

3. **Energy** balance between the Knee chakra and the posterior Sacral chakra at L4-L5 (Gov 3) through the hip joint.

4. Energy balance between the painful point on the hip and the Knee chakra until a change of emphasis is reached. This is often the most difficult and painstaking part of the procedure. Experience shows that patients experience chronic hip pain all around the hip and pelvic region, so trying to find a localized painful point can prove difficult—it's *all* painful! The only advice I can offer is to

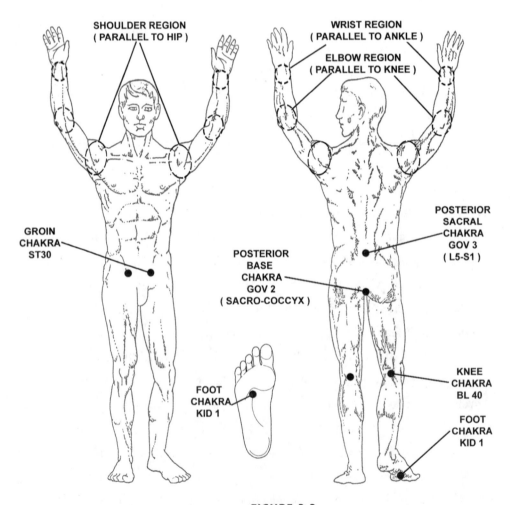

FIGURE 3.3

Points Used in the Treatment of Hip, Knee, and Ankle Conditions

use the points that are usually the most uncomfortable—these are the ones just behind the greater trochanter on the lateral aspect of the hip and the anterior aspect of the hip, which coincidentally relates to the Groin chakra at ST 30. The procedure of energy balancing needs to be done independently for both points.

5. Unwind the joint. This can be fun! You can do this in two ways: (a) with the hands placed on the anterior and posterior aspects of the joint and (b) with one hand on the lateral aspect at the greater trochanter and the other one around the upper part of the sacrum. Although you may perform the unwinding with the patient lying supine (a craniosacral therapist's nightmare!), the preferred position is lying on the side with the affected hip uppermost. Unwinding often takes a few minutes, and you must be prepared for sitting in the same position for a long time. Please see the final section of this chapter on the comfort of the therapist.

6. (a) Energy balance with the relative part of the shoulder joint on the same side of the body. (b) Energy balance with the same part of the opposite hip. (c) Energy balance with the posterior Sacral chakra and the Base chakra in the case of chronic arthritic changes. (d) Energy balance with the hip reflexes on the foot and arm (possibly on the hand).

Knee Joint

Conditions of the knee that therapists commonly encounter are acute sprains of the medial and lateral ligaments, torn cartilage or simple synovitis caused by repetitive strain (such as housemaids knee), and osteoarthritis. An osteoarthritic knee is very common and answers superbly to this type of treatment, as do subluxations or inflammation of the superior tibiofibular joint (STF syndrome).

Order of Treatment

(See Figure 3.3.)

1. Stroke the Kidney, Liver, and Spleen meridians (yin) from the toes toward the lower part of the abdomen and the Stomach, and the Gallbladder and Bladder meridians (yang) from the lower torso to the toes, that is, in the direction of energy flow.

2. Stimulate the Foot chakra on the sole of the foot (KID 1). Take care not to stimulate this point too much in patients with high blood pressure or in those who have a tendency to get headaches or circulation problems around the head or neck. Overstimulation could temporarily worsen these symptoms.

3. Energy balance between the Foot chakra and the Groin chakra (ST 30) through the knee joint lesion. It helps to visualize this, as explained earlier.

4. Energy balance between the painful part of the knee and the Foot chakra until a change of emphasis is attained. As with the previous example of the hip joint, there may be more than one pain point. In this case each one should be treated separately.

5. Unwind the joint. The anatomy of the knee joint lends itself easily to unwinding (a) with the hands placed on either side of the joint (laterally and medially) and (b) with the hands placed over the top and bottom of the joint (anteriorally and posteriorally).

6. (a) Energy balance between the lesion and the relevant part of the elbow on the same side of the body. (b) Energy balance between the lesion and exactly the same point on the other knee joint. (c) Energy balance between the lesion and the posterior Sacral chakra. It is also essential that the knee be balanced with the posterior Base chakra in every case of chronic condition. (d) Finally, energy balance between the lesion and the knee reflex on the foot and arm.

Ankle Joint

Ankle joint conditions that practitioners encounter range from an acute lateral sprain to osteoarthritis. Chronic Achilles tendonitis would also be treated using this method. As stated before, it is the chronic conditions that answer particularly well to this type of treatment—in other words, this approach works when others fail.

Order of Treatment

(See Figure 3.3.)

1. Stroke the same yin and yang meridians (channels) as you would for the Knee joint in the direction of the energy flow, but this time the strokes need only be between the toes and the hip area.

2. Stimulate the Foot chakra at KID 1.

3. Energy balance between the Foot chakra and the Knee chakra at BL 40 (middle of the popliteal fossa) through the lesion around the ankle.

4. Energy balance between the lesion (pain point) and the Foot chakra until a change of emphasis is attained. Please be aware that these two points may be very close to each other. This is particularly true in cases of metatarsalgia.

5. Unwind the joint. Again, the ankle lends itself to comfortable unwinding. Place the hands (a) on the anterior aspect of the joint and the Achilles area and (b) on the lateral and medial aspects of the ankle joint.

6. (a) Energy balance between the lesion and the appropriate region of the wrist on the same side of the body. In the case of metatarsalgia, use the metacarpal region. Feel for a tender point—you will find it! (b) Energy balance between the lesion and the same area on the opposite ankle joint. (c) Energy balance between the lesion

and the posterior Sacral chakra. Doing this hold successfully is particularly effective in the treatment of chronic ankle edema. Also balance between the lesion and the Base chakra in chronic conditions. (d) Finally, energy balance between the lesion and the reflexes found on the hand.

Other peripheral joints that may be treated are (a) the temporomandibular joint, (b) the sternoclavicular joint, (c) the symphysis pubis joint, and (d) the sacroiliac joint. Treatment of the temporomandibular and the sacroiliac joints will be covered later in the chapter under the section entitled "Case Histories." With regard to the other two, the same principles of treatment are used as with the limb joints.

SPINAL JOINT TREATMENT

Much about the basic treatment of spinal joints can be found in my book *Acupressure: Clinical Applications in Musculo-Skeletal Conditions,* yet there are many differences, both subtle and substantive, between treating purely with the chakra system and using generalized acupressure. This does not negate the use of general acupressure in the treatment of spinal conditions. Far from it; it simply means that an alternative approach seems to give faster and more lasting results.

Analysis and Assessment

There are literally scores of different spinal conditions. Each one gives a different set of signs and symptoms, and it would be impossible to cover each one individually. There is no need to, though, since the treatment of each follows the same procedure. Apart from some neurological conditions, it does not matter what diagnosis has been given to the problem, since the treatment—using chakra therapy—will be the same! Doctors and therapists often get bogged down in attempting to find a definitive diagnosis, which often isn't necessary. Of course, professional therapists have to use judgment and discernment with regard to conditions that fall outside their scope of clinical practice and expertise. If in doubt, do not tackle the problem, but hand the patient over to someone with the proper expertise. Although you may use chakra therapy to treat acute spinal conditions, they often answer very well to other forms of therapy, such as physical therapy, osteopathy, chiropractic, and acupuncture. It is, however, in the treatment of chronic spinal conditions that healing with the chakra energy system is the best type of hands-on therapy that you can use. I have used many different approaches with spinal conditions over a period of thirty-five years, so here I am speaking from much experience. All I ask is for you to try it—you will not be disappointed.

Acute Spinal Conditions

Acute conditions of any kind all present the same symptoms of pain (local and/or referred), muscle spasm, inflammation, and localized deformity. If not treated correctly during the first forty-eight hours after the lesion occurs, there is often a secondary effect of pain and acute deformity elsewhere in the spine, along with possible pain and stiffness in a peripheral joint. Examples of acute spinal lesions include:

- *Muscle tears* (to varying degrees) of the deep intravertebral muscles. These produce pain, localized inflammation, and swelling but rarely localized deformity.
- *Ligamentous tears* (to varying degrees) of the intervertebral ligaments. These produce pain, spasm, inflammation, and localized

deformity, resulting in the facet joint becoming subluxed or hyper-stretched.

- *Nerve-root inflammation.* This is caused by a sudden overstretch or lateral disc protrusion and produces very acute pain (local or radiating), localized muscle spasm, and inflammation. This can result in neuritis of the whole length of the inflamed nerve (e.g., sciatica).

- *Centralized disc protrusions.* These can cause excruciating localized and referred pain, spasm, and inflammation. Getting complete rest and taking anti-inflammatory medication are the only treatments initially, but using chakra acupressure after the first forty-eight hours helps wonderfully.

Often acute spinal lesions occur as a result of a chronic spinal weakness that may have been caused by a fall or some other trauma experienced as a child. The damage is done in infancy, and the person spends many years compensating for their underlying weakness. Eventually, during some activity (it does not have to be strenuous), the original weakness will give rise to acute symptoms.

Chronic Spinal Conditions

Examples of chronic spinal conditions include:

- *Muscular lesions.* These may occur as a result of a series of micro-traumas or because the spine attempts to compensate for an old postural imbalance. Microtraumas to the spine may be caused by repeated falling as a child or teenager either onto the coccyx region or onto the side (off a horse or fence, slipping on the ice, in the playground at school, etc). Old postural imbalances are caused by faulty posture as a child or teenager—slouching, sitting incorrectly for many hours at a time, getting insufficient exercise, or trying to compensate for being tall. There is usually local and distal pain, muscle spasm, lymphatic circulation inflammation, or congestion. Formations of fibrositic nodules within the muscles themselves sometimes form. This is called fibrositis or fibromyalgia as a generalized set of symptoms, or lumbago if occurring in the lumbar spine. Many doctors and therapists make light of fibrositis and quite often ignore lumbago as something that only occurred years ago. But these conditions are both very real.

- *Ligamentous lesions.* These are caused by old postural imbalances or as a result of repetitive overstretching of ligaments. Shortening and thickening of the interspinous ligaments occur, causing fixations of two or more vertebrae. The patient experiences diffuse pain and spasm, plus localized and distal deformity.

- *Chronic conditions following acute disc lesions* of the cervical and lumbar (occasionally thoracic) where there has been inadequate or no treatment during the acute phase. There will be multiple muscle spasms, ligamentous shortening and thickening, often fibrositic nodule formation, and a sluggish circulation of blood and lymph.

- *Congenital deformities* such as scoliosis, kyphosis, lordosis, and others. Although not always, these often result in symptoms later in life. There is usually a case, here, for gentle palliative treatment that eases pain and spasm, thus making everyday functions easier to perform. Vigorous therapy and surgical intervention may result in worse long-term prospects, at the expense of a more mobile spine.

- *Conditions resulting from surgical intervention,* for example, spinal fusion, laminectomy, discectomy, and so on. Chakra acupressure works very well for the ever-increasing number of patients in this category. You should realize, though, that the results you can achieve are only as good as the surgical intervention will allow.

Principles of Treatment

1. To reduce pain, inflammation, and deformity as much as is possible given the constrictions of the underlying anatomical deformity.
2. To increase the range of movement, thus reducing deformity.
3. To create an energy balance between the affected joint and its associations and correspondences in order to produce homoeostasis in the area.

Order of Treatment

The order of treatment is very similar to that used in the treatment of the peripheral joint conditions:

1. Massage around the affected area and the Bladder meridian.
2. Mobilize the vertebrae.
3. Stimulate the distal chakra point to create a reservoir of energy.
4. Balance energy *through* the affected vertebral region between the distal and the proximal chakra.
5. Balance energy between the spinal lesion and the distal chakra.
6. Balance the joint with its coupled reflexes—Parallel, Minor, Foot, and Hand chakras.
7. Unwind the joint.
8. Finally mobilize or adjust the joint accordingly.

Explanation of Treatment

1. A practical hands-on therapist need not be convinced of the positive advantages of massage in all its forms. On top of the physiological improvements to the circulation of blood and lymph, the

psychological boost is also very important. Never underestimate the power of touch on the psyche. Patients generally feel more comfortable when hands are placed on them. The following types of massage are needed:

a. *Generalized soothing massage.* Initially you have to feel the patient's tissues, and they need to appreciate your hands. It is a two-way dialogue. Just do a few short and long strokes of effleurage (preferably using soya oil) along the whole length of the spine. This is soothing to the patient and also allows you to learn about the state of the tissues.

b. *Local massage.* Massage around the lesion with a few short strokes of effleurage or finger and thumb pad kneading. It is also possible to do some short strokes of connective tissue massage (CTM). Please warn the patient before you perform CTM, since it can be quite sharp. CTM is a wonderful form of massage that improves the blood and lymphatic circulation and is well worth learning if you have not learned it already.

c. *Bladder meridian massage.* This is performed using the pads of the middle and index fingers, placed on either side of the spine, massaging with fairly heavy pressure from the neck down to the sacral region. The "inner" bladder line extends more laterally from the spine at the lumbar end than it does at the cervical, and the spread of the fingers should accommodate this difference. With chronic spinal conditions, you will need to improve the energetic quantity in the local and distal areas of the spine, and massaging the bladder meridian is one way of doing this. The use of CTM along the inner and outer bladder lines is particularly effective in the lumbosacral region. Following the massage, the affected area should be a little more hyperemic and relaxed.

2. Next, the affected vertebra should be gently mobilized in order to stretch the tight ligaments and to further improve localized blood flow. Physical therapists should be well versed in Maitland mobilizing, the perfect form of mobilizing in this instance. For those of you not trained in this procedure, the spinous processes of the affected vertebrae need to be gently pushed from posterior to anterior (P-A movement) with the patient lying prone. You may perform this with the thumb pads or the heel of the hand using the pisiform bone. The vertebrae should be mobilized with short repetitive thrust movements for up to thirty seconds per vertebra by very gentle pressure just enough to visibly move the joint. This represents no more than Maitland Grade 2 mobilizing. It is *not* manipulation!

3. So far, this approach has involved the usual way in which a physical therapist may commence the treatment of a spinal condition. The difference in this method starts here. The distal chakra point needs to be stimulated in order to create a reservoir of energy (chi) within the spine. This is an imperative stage in the treatment of chronic conditions. There is no way that chronic conditions may be addressed without some stimulation of energy. Chronic conditions usually come with sluggish and congested tissues, and the energy within has to be stimulated. Success needs to be worked toward. Although it is true that the Base chakra needs to be stimulated in every chronic spinal condition, it is only necessary to do this in chronic forms of spinal arthritis such as cervical, thoracic, and lumbar spondylosis. This can be done as well as the one that is normally indicated—this will be explained later in the section about the treatment of individual spinal areas. The distal chakra point needs to be stimulated with the finger pad for at

least two minutes until a detectable change of heat and "point pliability" is felt. If you are unsure as to how long the stimulation needs to be done, stop it for a few seconds to see if the point feels different. If you feel no discernible sensation, then stimulate for another minute or so (yes, it's a long time) and then hold again for a few seconds. Repeat this stimulate-hold routine for as long as it takes to achieve a definite difference in the tissues immediately around the point. With a severe spinal arthritis, for example, it could take as long as five to six minutes before this occurs. It is always a good thing to "overdo" the stimulating massage of the distal chakra point—there is more chi to use for the later work, and it cannot be overdone.

4. The next stage is to energy balance between the distal chakra point that has just been stimulated and the proximal chakra point. It may be that an energy balance will be reached after only half a minute or so, but it usually takes a lot longer than that. The object of the exercise is to stimulate and energize *through* the lesion. In acute conditions, this will occur after a few seconds; in chronic ones it will take a lot longer. The proximal chakra point will also have to be stimulated, along with the distal point. Both the therapist and the patient will note that by now the spine will be feeling generally more relaxed even though seemingly there has been no specific work performed on the lesion.

5. Now is the time to finally place the hands on the lesion. Though it is a personal preference, I prefer to treat upper cervical lesions with the patient supine and the remainder of the spine (lower cervical to coccyx) with him or her prone lying with access to an adequate "breathing" hole in the couch. With cervical lesions it is easier to place a finger pad on the lesion while balancing with the

opposite finger pad under the distal chakra point. For lesions further down the spine it becomes a matter of choice. The whole hand or just the finger pad may be used to give localized pressure. Do whatever feels most comfortable.

As with the treatment of peripheral joints, this part of the procedure is most important and requires total focus on your part. The hold must be continued until a change of energy emphasis has taken place. Immediately after this occurs, both you and the patient will feel an immediate sensation of relief within the lesion area. you will feel as if a "breakthrough" has been made. In reality, this is not far from the truth—from this point on, the therapist may energy balance the lesion with other points just to "strengthen" the healing that has occurred and to enable the therapy done so far to be reinforced.

6. This is achieved by energy balancing the lesion with its various correspondences and associations. These are (a) the corresponding spinal point according to the Lovett brother association, that is, C1 to L5, C2 to L4, and so on. Please note that this is not the spinal "harmonic" of polarity therapy. (b) The associated reflex on the foot or hand (which depends on comfort and ease of access) (c) the adjacent minor chakra(s).

7. Now it is time to unwind the joint. There are three ways to do this—only one need be carried out, but the treatment will be enhanced if all three are completed. (a) The easiest way is to place the hands either side of the lesion, proximally and distally to the lesion on the spine (b) Or you can place your hands on either side the lesion, laterally to the spine. In these first two approaches the gap between the hands is minimal (about one 1 inch) (c) You can also place one hand over the lesion and the other over the Lovett

brother vertebra previously discovered. In this case, there is sometimes quite a distance between the two hands. In all three ways of unwinding, the principle and procedure are the same. For the first minute or so after placing your hands on the patient, there will be little or no reaction. Slowly and gradually, though, the tissues under your hands will appear to move and change their texture with the tissues appearing to relax and becoming warmer as it happens. Please do not oppose any of the unwinding; the whole principle is to "go with it." When the unwinding has been completed, the next stage can be commenced. It is, though, impossible to completely unwind a forty-year-old old lesion in one attempt. The body is, of course, very wise and will only unwind as far as it is meant to in a particular treatment session.

8. The joint and its immediate area will now be feeling very much more pliable and relaxed than before. The treatment session can finish now, or you may further mobilize the offending vertebrae to further increase the ligamentous elasticity and also to check that there really is more vertebral movement than there was.

TREATMENT OF SPECIFIC SPINAL LEVELS

This section deals with the many aspects of treating muscle conditions the chakra energy system.

Cervical Spine C1-C4

(See Figure 3.4.)

The patient should be supine with his or her head supported on a single pillow—or preferably on a "bean" bag. This will allow plenty of room for your hands and fingers to slide under the neck, and it will be more comfortable for the patient. It is possible to treat the patient in prone position with his or her face in a suitable comfortable breathing hole, but the supine position seems to give more control and is certainly more patient friendly.

This region of the neck is often affected by stress-related conditions. The modern pace of life produces tension in the neck, which in turn creates muscle spasm and localized inflammation. This affects the nerve flow in the region as well as the cerebrospinal fluid flow, which in turn may give rise to strain in the eyes, catarrh, ear tension, headaches, dizziness, and head fullness. Chakra acupressure and bodywork are admirably suited to easing these symptoms.

Order of Treatment

1. The general region should be massaged with a little oil (this is a preference). This massage should consist of some general effleurage and stroking. It is then important to knead the paravertebral muscles that may or may not be in spasm. This automatically means that the Bladder meridian is massaged. The massage should take a couple of minutes and should be long enough to relax the patient and to ascertain the lesion site.

2. Mobilize the spinous processes and the transverse processes (if you are competent to do so) of C1-C4, making a note of where there is restriction of movement, pain, and so forth.

3. The distal chakra point is the posterior Throat chakra at C7-T1 (Gov 14). This should be stimulated for about a minute or until the point feels warm and "full of energy." As stated earlier, with any kind of chronic spinal condition, the Base chakra should also be stimulated, especially in osteoarthritic conditions. It is not essen-

tial to treat the posterior Base chakra; just stimulate whichever point is easiest to get at. The anterior Base chakra at Con 2 (just proximal to the symphysis pubis) is the point of ease with the patient lying on her back, whereas the posterior Base chakra point at Gov 2 (sacrococcyx junction) would be stimulated if they she is lying prone. The cardinal rule in both examples is to inform the patient before you touch him/her and to seek his/her permission.

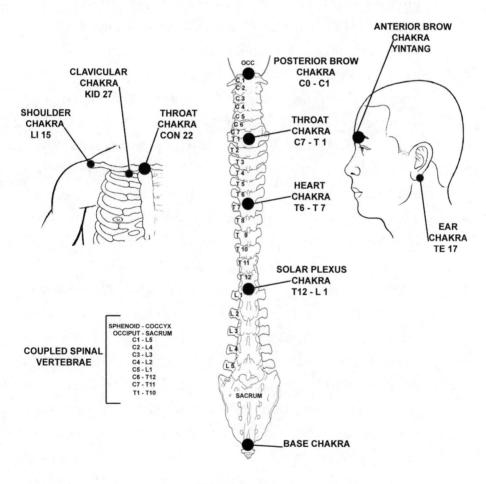

FIGURE 3.4

Points Used in Cervical Spine Conditions

Both chakra points are situated in a very vulnerable part of the anatomy, and it is always politic to enquire. Simply say, "Is it OK if I put my hand here?" or something along those lines.

4. The next step is to energy balance between the distal chakra point (posterior Throat chakra) and the posterior Brow chakra, situated at the inion just distal to the occiput (C0-C1). If the lesion is close to the atlas or occiput, it is best to make the Crown chakra the proximal point. The point of the exercise is to energy balance *through* the lesion. In very chronic conditions, I suggest that you stimulate both points and hold them for a few seconds, repeated a few times before the balance is attained.

5. Place one middle finger pad on the lesion site and the other middle finger pad on the posterior Throat chakra (where it has been all this time). This is the most important aspect of the treatment session, and the two points should be held until a change of emphasis is felt (maybe about three minutes or so).

6. Now energy balance with the various adjacent points and correspondences to augment the treatment. The adjacent points are: (a) both Ear chakra points at TE 17, (b) both Shoulder chakra points at LI 15, (c) both Clavicular chakra points at KID 27, (d) the anterior Throat chakra (Con 22), and (e) the anterior Brow chakra at Extra 1 (Yintang).

The correspondences are: (a) the parallel zone, or Lovett Brother, of C1-L5; C2-L4; C3-L3; C4-L2. The hand will have to be gently placed under the patient's back if he is lying supine. The easy way to do this is to place the whole hand over the area of the lesion and the other hand underneath the L2-L5 region. (b) If possible, balance the lesion with the reflex on the hand and/or foot (c) When your patient is suffering from referred pain or parasthesia (pins and needles) down the arm, it is very helpful to balance the lesion with the Elbow chakra (P3) and the Hand chakra (P8)

7. The penultimate stage is to unwind the lesion or area. This area presents quite a challenge in unwinding, but it may be achieved successfully by one of three methods. Why not do them all?: (a) Place the middle finger pads both sides of the spinous process (virtually over the transverse process) and push into the tissues very gently. After a few seconds the lesion will appear to unwind as you fingers go "with the flow." This may go on for a couple of minutes or so. (b) Place the hand (maybe just two or three fingers because of lack of space) on either side above and below the lesion area. (c) Place one hand over the whole lesion area and the other hand over the parallel zone area (L2-L5). This procedure could be done at the same time as the parallel balancing was done in the previous section. Unwinding in this case may be quite severe. Do not be surprised if your patient seems almost to want to come off the couch as the muscles start to let go and unwind.

8. The final stage is to check the range of movement in the region either by mobilizing or stretching the area yourself or to ask the patient to do it in a series of requested head movements. He or she may be very surprised at the results!

Cervical Spine C5, C6, and C7-T1

(See Figure 3.4.)

This area represents a very "busy" one in the spine, it being the center of parallelogram of forces down the spine and across to the shoulders and arms. Many chronic lesions occur here, such as cervical spondylosis and disc lesions, which often give referred pain down the arm, the back of the shoulder blade, or the front of the chest. Chakra acupressure and bodywork can be very rewarding to those with these disabling and painful conditions. This region of the neck may be treated with the patient prone or supine. Most practitioners prefer prone treatment, and if this is the case, make sure the patient has a comfortable, well-padded breathing hole. Never attempt to treat a cervical spine in prone unless there is a breathing hole so that the patient's head is not turned to the side.

Order of Treatment

1. Massage the local area and also perform some long and short strokes along the paravertebral region, across to the shoulders and down the arms. Finger pad kneading can also be done down the Bladder meridian. CTM is extremely effective in this region, especially with chronic conditions where there may be more than a few deposits of fibrositic nodules.

2. It is important to mobilize the vertebrae in this region, as described earlier. As well as offering a service to the patient in treating the area, this procedure also gives you an opportunity to assess where the lesions or the sore points are.

3. There is a choice of distal chakras to stimulate. In chronic conditions, the Base chakra has to be stimulated, regardless of what else is done. The posterior Heart chakra (T6-T7) should be stimulated if there is much tension in the region due to an obvious emotional history, but the posterior Solar Plexus chakra (T12-L1) is the one of choice if there is not an emotional history. It is either/or with these two, but in the case of chronic conditions stimulate the Base chakra point as well. The rest of the treatment, including the energy balancing, will be carried out with the Heart or Solar

Plexus. The stimulation of either point last be for over two minutes, in the same manner as described previously.

4. The next stage is to energy balance between the posterior Heart/posterior Solar Plexus and the proximal chakra of the posterior Brow just below the occiput (C0-C1). Try and visualize the energy flowing *through* the lesion.

5. Now energy balance between the lesion itself and the posterior Heart/Solar Plexus chakra point. This is the most important stage of the treatment and needs to be held until a change of emphasis is ascertained. If there is more than one sore point, both need to be balanced with the distal chakra point.

6. The lesion now needs to be energy balanced with all the local and distal reflected points in order to support the preceding part of the treatment. The adjacent points are: Adjacent points (a) both Shoulder chakra points at LI 15, (b) the anterior Throat chakra points at Con 22, (c) both Clavicular chakra points at KID 27, and (d) both Elbow chakra points at PC 8, if there is any referred pain to the elbows.

   The correspondences are: (a) the parallel zone of T10-L1. Instead of localizing the exact lesion, it is enough to place the whole hand over the lesion and balance it with the area T10-L1. This gives an amazingly good energy balance. (b) Balance with the reflected point on the foot or hand. The patient may be taught to use the hand reflex especially in home treatment.

7. Now is the time to unwind the lesion. This can be performed in one of several ways. As before, try them all! (a) Place the middle finger pads, supported by the adjacent fingers on either side of the spine at the level of the lesion, approximately two inches lateral to the midline. This unwinding is best performed with the

patient in supine but can be done in prone (b) The better way is to unwind by placing the whole hand either side of the spine at the lesion level (c) Place the whole hand distally and proximally to the lesion (d) Place one hand over the lesion and the other hand over the parallel region of T10-L1. (e) Please note that there is another unwinding procedure—to unwind between the lesion area and the anterior Throat chakra. This will be discussed in the chapter on healing, since it has more significant ramifications than just treating musculoskeletal conditions.

8. Now the region needs to be finally mobilized so that you can ascertain the improvement of the region and iron out any residual problems in the tissues. Please check the patient's range of movement when he or she sits up.

Thoracic Spine

(See Figure 3.5.)

The whole of the thoracic spine will be discussed in this section because the distal and proximal points used are the same. Each vertebral level, though, may exhibit different symptoms apart from the usual ones of pain and spasm. Owing to the existence of the sympathetic chain of nerves (that form part of the autonomic nervous system) lying alongside the transverse processes, a lesion at different levels may give rise to different internal organ system. You need not be too concerned about individual symptoms, though; just to be aware that internal organic imbalance could be caused by thoracic spinal lesions—and vice versa.

Order of Treatment

1. First do some massage so as to improve the circulation of the area.

This may be accomplished by giving some long and short stroke effleurage on either side of the spine, massaging along the costal margins and intercostals spaces between the ribs, and kneading along the inner Bladder meridian line.

2. Next mobilize the vertebrae around the lesion. It is better to mobilize the vertebrae that are most distal from the lesion first and then to home in on the affected vertebral level. Doing it this way

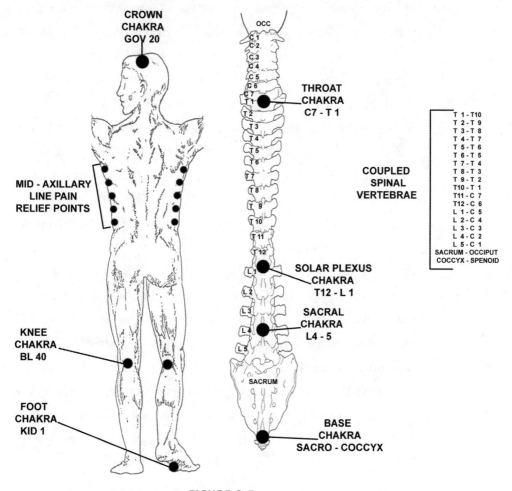

FIGURE 3.5
Points Used in Thoracic, Lumbar, and Sacrococcyx Conditions

will give you a better indication of where the exact lesion lies. Scoliosis of the spine often affects the thoracic spine. This condition is quite varied and is often congenital, and nothing really to worry about unless it is giving symptoms either locally or around the ribs to the front of the body. If it is a rotoscoliosis where there is some vertebral body misalignment or "collapse," this could give direct discomfort to the stomach/diaphragm region as well as giving ANS symptoms. In the case of fixation of some of the thoracic vertebrae due to either an "S" curve or a long "C" curve, these are obviously not going to respond to mobilization. I believe that *any* movement is better than none at all and that even spinal fixations should be encouraged to move a little. *Movement is life!*

3. Now it is time to stimulate the distal chakra point in order to create a reservoir of energy in the spine. This is the posterior Sacral chakra at L4-5. In the case of chronic conditions, do not forget also to stimulate the Base chakra. The two may be stimulated at the same time with a rhythmical stimulate-hold pattern until you are certain that a change in the tissues has taken place.

4. Balance the posterior Sacral chakra with the proximal chakra point, which is the posterior Throat chakra at Gov 14 (C7-T1). Be certain to visualize energy flowing *through* the lesion area. This should be done for about two minutes or until there is a sensation of oneness underneath the finger pads.

5. Now find the lesion and energy balance with this point and the posterior Sacral chakra. As stated before, this is the most important aspect of the treatment; if this part is not done correctly the whole treatment will fall short of the expected outcome. A change of emphasis *has* to occur in this part of the treatment.

6. Now it is time to energy balance the lesion with the adjacent and

correspondent reflexes. Since the condition lies within the thoracic spine, it is unlikely that there will be a parallel zonal area with which to balance unless the lesion is at, say, T2 when that would be balanced with T9. The closer the lesion lies to the "fulcrum" part of the spine at T6-T7, the less likely it will be that a parallel point will be found due to the proximity of the hands. There are two reflected areas, though, that are very useful. One is the thoracic reflex on the foot and the other "set" of reflexes found on the axillary line (lateral aspect of the chest). From the lesion, wherever it may be, follow the rib around to its outer aspect and balance with the point there. This point will always be tender, since it is the reflected point of the lesion.

7. Unwinding is very comforting and rewarding in all thoracic conditions. It may be performed in the way previously described, with the exception of omitting the parallel area. Unwinding is best done with the whole hand on either side of the spine followed by the whole of the hand proximal and distal to the lesion.

8. Now remobilize the region so as to reinforce the previous work and to treat any individual residual concern that was not discovered previously. Please also note that in chronic conditions, it is impossible to treat every symptom in just one session; you may need several.

Lumbar Spine

(See Figure 3.5.)

This region of the spine takes most of the body weight, and is therefore subject to more strain than any other part of the body (apart from the ball of the foot). It is therefore not surprising that bodyworkers spend more patient-hours treating this area than any other. Lumbar spinal conditions cause as many sick days in the Western world as the common cold. Treating chronic lumbar conditions can be extremely rewarding when using chakra acupressure. The conditions that you are most likely to encounter are acute lumbar pain (due to a myriad of reasons), acute or chronic sciatica, osteoarthritis of the lumbar spine, and sequela prolapsed intervertebral disc (PID).

Order of Treatment

1. The whole region needs to be massaged so as to improve the local circulation and to enable the tissues to become more pliable and comfortable. This may be done by performing short and long effleurage strokes, by giving finger pad massage along the Bladder meridian, and by thumb or finger pad kneading to the areas that are most sluggish. CTM is extremely beneficial when carried out in this region of the spine.

2. Now mobilize the lumbar vertebrae with Maitland mobilizing or something similar. This is an excellent way to start the process of movement of the vertebrae as well as being the ideal way to ascertain the exact lesion point or area. Spend at least a minute doing this.

3. Next stimulate the distal chakra point, which is the posterior Base chakra (sacrococcyx). In very chronic and long-standing lumbar conditions, this needs to be done for about four to five minutes before an obvious difference is felt under the finger pad. Don't give up after three minutes if there is seemingly no change—it *will* happen. You must have patience when dealing with these conditions. When treating acute lumbar spinal conditions the stimulation will take far less time. Remember that the point of doing this is to create a reservoir of energy in the spine that can be used later. There are *no* short cuts when using this type of chakra system.

4. The distal chakra point is now balanced with the proximal chakra point, which is the posterior Solar Plexus chakra point at T12-L1. If the lesion happens to be a rare one at L1, then the posterior Heart chakra should be used as the proximal point. With chronic conditions, both the distal and proximal points need to be stimulated together, and it may take as long as three to four minutes before an energy balance is achieved *through* the lesion. Visualization and focus on the job in hand are essential at this stage.

5. Now is the time to energy balance the lesion with the posterior Base chakra. Since the lumbar vertebrae are much larger than the cervical or thoracic, the actual lesion site may not be directly over the spinous or transverse processes, but slightly lateral to the transverse process in the musculature of the erector spinae muscle. This would be true in many cases of sciatica. There may be several "ouch" points and each need to be balanced in turn. During this part of the treatment, it is vital that a change of emphasis is felt. Failure to do so would generally negate the rest of the treatment.

6. The lesion now has to be energy balanced with the adjacent points and the correspondent reflexes. The adjacent points are: (a) posterior Solar Plexus chakra, (b) the posterior Sacral point if the lesion is L1/2, (c) the Knee chakra, especially in sciatica, and (d) the Foot chakra, especially in sciatica.

    The Correspondences are: (a) the foot reflex, a very useful tool especially in pain relief and (b) the parallel zone area of the cervical area, which is also extremely useful. Remember that the couples are L5 with C1, L4 with C2, L3 with C3, L2 with C4, and L1 with C5. Performing this balance with the middle finger pads allows you to be specific. This leads nicely to the next stage.

7. Now the lesion needs to be unwound. This may be done in three different ways. If time permits, it is best to use all three methods, since the patient will benefit greatly. While the fingers are placed on the lesion and zone area of the cervical spine, change the position slightly by placing the whole hand over the lesion and the other hand over the neck, and proceed to unwind. There may not be any obvious movement at first, but after about half a minute the hands will appear to respond to the changes in the tissues beneath. As stated before, the golden rule in unwinding is to go with the flow and never to oppose the body's natural movement. You are merely the facilitator, not the "doer." The other ways to unwind are to place the hands on either side of the spine; you can also place them just proximally and distally to the lesion.

8. Now mobilize the lumbar spine again. You will find that there is much more pain-free movement in the area than there was before the treatment commenced, as will your patient when he or she is finally off the couch.

Sacrum and Coccyx

(See Figure 3.5.)

The sacrum represents the foundation or basement of the building, the remainder of the vertebrae being the other floors. It is therefore imperative to have a stable foundation, otherwise the floors will get out of alignment, and mechanical lesions will ensue. Many practitioners believe that the sacrum should be treated with *any* chronic vertebral lesion. This area represents just two aspects of the spine, but they are hugely disparate in size, and the ensuing symptoms are very different. These could be sacroiliitis, sacroiliac subluxations or fixation, spinal scoliosis, sciatica, hemorrhoids, coccydinia, and foot pain. There is nothing more miserable for someone than to endure the agony of acute or chronic coccydinia or even a displacement of the bone after falling heavily onto the base of the spine. This often happens when some "clown" (the word is chosen carefully, since these people cannot be cursed enough) pulls away a chair that a poor unfortunate is just about to sit on. Even though the coccyx is a small, seemingly insignificant bone, the ramifications of a lesion at the base of the spine can be enormous. There is nowhere for the resultant inflammation and bruising to go, and since the region is acutely sore, the person does not want it to be touched. It may slowly resolve when the patient sits on ice packs for a few days, followed by receiving gentle rehabilitation.

Order of Treatment

1. Massage the area thoroughly, including the Bladder meridian. It is worth spending a few extra moments doing some thumb or finger pad kneading in the sacral foramen. CTM is particularly effective in this area. Try also to massage the ileotibial tracts of both thighs. This region is called the lymphatic congestion area of the lower lumbar spine. In every case of lumbosacral insufficiency and chronic pain, the lymphatic drainage of the area becomes sluggish. This in turn creates lymphatic deposits along the outside of the thighs. This area is very painful when massaged, and the patient must be warned in advance. In the case of coccydinia, massage is not required.

2. Now the sacrum and/or coccyx needs to be mobilized with Maitland mobilizing or something similar. Take care when mobilizing the sacroiliac joints in the case of sciatica and of mobilizing the sacrococcygeal joint in the case of coccydinia.

3. Now the distal chakra point needs to be stimulated. This is the posterior Base chakra at the sacrococcygeal junction for sacral conditions and either the Knee or Foot chakra when dealing with coccyx problems. These points need to be stimulated for about two to three minutes in the case of long-standing conditions or until a definite alteration in the feel of the tissue is felt.

4. Now balance between the distal chakra point and the proximal chakra point, which is the posterior Sacral chakra at L4-5. This is to move energy *through* the lesion. As stated before, this process is reinforced by visualization and focus.

5. Now find the lesion point or area and balance the sore point of the lesion with the distal chakra point. In the case of chronic sacrum or coccyx lesions, the hold/stimulation should proceed until a change of emphasis is achieved. In the case of acute sacroiliac or coccyx lesions, take care not to press on the point too hard, or it may become too painful for the patient. In these cases, place the finger very gently on the point and allow the heat and inflammation to disperse through your fingers. As it does, your fingers will be able to press a little deeper. When dealing with all coccyx conditions, you must inform your patient when he or she is about to be touched there and to verbally seek permission. It may be difficult to attain a change of emphasis in very acute conditions.

6. Now balance the lesion with the adjacent chakra points and the corresponding reflexes. The adjacent points are: (a) the posterior Sacral chakra at L4-5 and (b) the Knee chakra at BL 40. The correspondences are: (a) the sacrum's parallel zone region is the occiput. The whole hand needs to be placed over the occiput, even though a tender point/area will be found to match the lesion on the sacrum. The coccyx corresponds with the Crown chakra point

at Gov 20. This point just needs to be held in the case of acute coccyx conditions and stimulated in the case of hemorrhoids or other
chronic pelvic conditions. This approach works wonders! (b) The
foot reflex is a very useful adjunct in the case of pain.

7. Unwinding is an extremely useful tool and may be performed in
   one of two ways. The first way is to place the hands on either side
   of the sacrum around the bilateral sacroiliac region. The second
   way is to place one whole hand on the sacrum and the other on the
   occiput. Unwinding of the coccyx can only be performed with the
   one hold of the lesion and the Crown chakra at Gov 20.

8. Finally, mobilize the area again to further increase the range of
   movement within these not-too-moveable joints.

The therapist using just acupressure and bodywork based on the
chakra energy system should have enough knowledge about the
points suggested to achieve the desired results. There are, though,
a few more types of acupressure energy balancing, and these could
be useful adjuncts when looking at the whole package being offered.
These will be discussed fully in my book *The Holistic Spine*.

THE THERAPIST'S COMFORT

I have included this short section since the topic of staying comfortable applies to therapists who do bodywork, acupressure, reflexology, and healing. Although this area is often overlooked by
practitioners, it is vitally important. It is often difficult for therapists
to admit that they are just as prone to the conditions described in
his book—lower back pain, neck strain, headaches, repetitive stress
syndrome, and general tension—as anyone else. With this type of

work, you will often find yourself in lengthy sessions that consist of just holding two points, sometimes with outstretched arms, so it is imperative that you take every opportunity to relax into the treatment. It will help you to observe the following safeguards:

1. Sit down whenever it is practical to do so.

2. Invest in a "wheely" chair, thus making it easier to treat the patient and to go from one set of holding points to the next without having to stand up or move the chair. Also try to use a hydraulic couch so that you may adjust the height. Although these are more expensive than portable couches, they are worth the investment. If you work out of your home, it might also be more difficult for you to use one of these.

3. When holding two points with either finger or hands, don't be afraid to ask the patient if you can rest your forearms on him or her, thus relieving the tension in your shoulders, neck, and arms. Usually patients will not mind at all. Also try to support your forearms on the couch whenever possible.

4. Between treatments, get up and walk around or do some neck and lower back stretching exercises.

5. Hygiene demands that you wash your hands between patients. Although the type of healing you are practicing has nothing to do with spiritual healing or the laying on of hands, you might encounter some patients who exude negative "vibes," so it is always best to safeguard yourself by washing your hands in cold running water (cold water is generally purer than hot).

6. Finally, learn to relax into the therapy. This is difficult to do while you are still learning but will become easier the more experienced you become. Enjoy it!

Because I have always found that practical workbooks containing case histories of real patients make the subject at hand more believable and acceptable, to that end I have included several in the next section.

ACUPRESSURE AND BODYWORK CASE HISTORIES

I have included these four case histories to give you a better understanding of how you can use this type of therapy. I have chosen to use case studies of former patients, all of whom have consented to their stories being told here.

Lower Back Pain with Sciatica (and Atlas Involvement)

History

David was a twenty-five-year-old motor mechanic who even at this tender age was suffering from what he and his general physician considered a repetitive strain of the lumbar spine, brought on by his constantly adopting a posture of being bent over while leaning over car hoods. He had suffered a previous episode of lower back pain at age sixteen when he fell heavily on the ice. This resulted in a bruised coccyx (and pride) but seemingly little else. It was also ascertained that he suffered from occasional neck strain and from fairly constant headaches over the eyes. The latter symptom was probably caused by a misaligned atlas/axis brought on by a heavy fall. He also had irritable bowel syndrome, which was both painful and embarrassing for him.

Examination

The examination revealed a rotation of the atlas (right), tightness in the cervical and thoracic spine, lumbar 5 rotation (left), L5-S1 facet joint lock (left), a very tight sacroiliac joint (left), and an obvious left fixation of the coccyx. There was also an apparent short leg (left) of approximately a half-inch. This became the "long" leg when his knees were flexed. Although he could have been treated using a more conventional type of physical therapy, we decided to use chakra acupressure and bodywork, since David presented a multitude of problems. Using traditional treatment would have subjected him to more treatment, and his limited budget needed to be taken into account.

First Treatment Session

1. Since David's short leg altered when his knees were flexed, this indicated that there was an atlas involvement (merely verification of other symptoms). The first thing to do was to adjust the leg-length differential. This was achieved by placing the middle finger pads on the Hand chakra and Foot chakra on the long leg side, creating an instant adjustment.

2. We decided to concentrate on the painful lumbosacral region and sciatica in the first session, so I administered some massage and mobilizing. This work also indicated that there was L5-S1 (left) tension. Since David was only twenty-five and had had the condition for a relatively short period, the surrounding joints were quite mobile, it was very easy to identify the lesion and the "ouch" point.

3. I stimulated the Base chakra at the sacrococcygeal junction for about two minutes. It did not take long for the heat to build up under the

fingers and for the underlying tissues to become more pliant. David remarked that the area was beginning to feel more relaxed.

4. I then energy balanced the Base chakra with the Sacral chakra (proximal chakra). This did not take long, since there was already quite a lot of "energy" in the region.

5. The lesion (over the left transverse process of L5) was located and energy balanced with the Base chakra until a change of emphasis was produced—very effective in pain relief.

6. The lesion was then energy balanced with the foot reflex, the Foot chakra, and the Knee chakra on the left leg. At first the sciatic pain seemed to increase slightly (not unusual) before it eased.

7. I then unwound the lesion by placing my hands over its lateral aspects, and also by balancing it with the parallel point of the atlas. After that, I placed one whole hand over the lesion and the other on the occipital/upper-cervical region. This proved very effective, and I needed to hold my hands in place for about five minutes while all the preceding muscular tension unwound and relaxed.

8. During the final mobilizing, the L5-S1 facet joint seemed to "give" quite easily (spontaneous adjustment) with no undue pressure whatsoever. David then stood up, and when I asked him to walk, flex, and side-flex his spine to see how it felt, he reported that it was much better.

Second Treatment Session

I saw David one week later, and he showed much less discomfort in the lower spine and leg, although he was still on sick leave and had not "properly worked" his back. He had still been experiencing recurrent headaches and a "cotton wool" sensation in his head behind the eyes (cranial base etiology). Examination revealed that there was much less spasm/pain/inflammation in the lower lumbar spine. David felt sciatic pain just outside the knee joint. There was no leg-length differential. The atlas seemed tight, although there was no appreciable misalignment.

1. I massaged and mobilized David's lower back. This was followed by massage of the Bladder meridian from the lumbar all the way up to the cranium, with David in the prone position.

2. I then stimulated the posterior Base chakra so as to create a reservoir of energy within the whole spine. This was quickly followed by energy balancing the Base to the Sacral chakra through the lumbar lesion. The lesion was then balanced with the Base chakra until a change of emphasis was reached. The whole area was now much more comfortable.

3. The lumbar lesion was balanced with the left Knee chakra so as to ease the remaining sciatic referral. This was achieved with ease. The lumbar spine was finally mobilized.

4. I now turned my attention to the remaining lesion at the upper cervical area. Since there was already lots of energy in the spinal complex, the first stage was to energy balance through the lesion by holding the posterior Throat chakra and the Crown chakra. I decided that the posterior Brow chakra was not the proximal point, since it was too close to the lesion. The lesion was found to be the right transverse process of the atlas. This was balanced with the posterior Throat chakra until a change of emphasis was achieved.

5. I then energy balanced the lesion with the Shoulder chakras, anterior Brow chakra, Ear chakras, and Clavicular chakras. It was while I was balancing with the anterior Brow chakra that the facet joint of C0-C1 seemed to "give" as a spontaneous release—this is often due to the relaxation of the tissues.

6. I placed both sets of fingers on either side of the lesion to help it unwind. Finally, the area was balanced with the lower lumbar spine. After the joint was gently mobilized, David sat up and carefully moved his head and neck to check for pain and limitation of movement. Most of the discomfort seemed to have disappeared. He was due back at work the following day, so I taught him some neck and lower back strengthening exercises and told him to contact me if he needed any more therapy.

David telephoned one week later, reporting that he had had a great week with no pain and a full range of movement. He was still doing his exercises to strengthen his back extensors. The irritable bowel syndrome had also been much improved.

It is not uncommon to be able to treat a fairly complex spinal condition in just two sessions. If, however, David had been twenty to thirty years older and the lesions had been more chronic, an extra session or two would have been required.

Osteoarthritis of the Knee
History

Daisy was a fifty-five-year-old farmer's wife who had worked hard all her life. She had osteoarthritis changes in both knees (she brought the X-rays with her), although just the right one was giving her trouble. She had started to feel pain over eighteen months earlier, and she had received physical therapy as well as analgesics and anti-inflammatory medication. Daisy had been referred by her next-door neighbor (a regular patient) and was very skeptical. She told me that she had fallen several times over the years, landing on her back and knees but had endured no other previous injuries. Her right ankle was painful and swollen, and her lower spine had given her trouble off and on for the past twenty years. Although I probed regarding the state of her emotional and mental health, she was not forthcoming. I then decided to treat the problem as a purely musculoskeletal condition and to observe her responses as the treatment progressed.

Examination

Both knees were quite swollen and indurated. The right one was hot and inflamed to the touch. Flexion and hyperextension were restricted, but normal cruciate movement was elicited. The weight-bearing "line" was badly out on the right foot, and Daisy had quite a lot of hard skin on the soles of both feet.

First Treatment Session

1. We decided to concentrate on the knee in the first session and not to attempt to treat the lower spine. Daisy lay supine on the couch, with just her legs exposed. I began treatment with some massage using long strokes along the meridian lines and short strokes around the knee; I also employed some passive movements to the knee and to both feet (especially to the metatarsal joints in order to free them up a little and to improve the circulation generally).

2. I decided to stimulate the Knee chakra first (the center of the popliteal fossa at BL 40) in order to improve local circulation. I then stimulated the distal chakra point of the Foot chakra (KID 1) on the right foot. It took considerable time before the tissues felt more yielding. I followed by energy balancing between the Foot chakra and the anterior Base chakra in an attempt to draw energy through the knee.

3. The focal point of the knee was the joint margin just lateral to the

quadriceps tendon. I held and balanced this point with the Foot chakra until a change of emphasis was felt. At this point, Daisy suddenly told me that the tension and tightness in her knee had suddenly eased. I carried on the hold for longer than usual until the lesion itself was balanced with other points. These were the opposite Knee chakra, the Elbow chakra on the same side, and the anterior Sacral chakra at acupoint Con 6.

4. Unwinding the knee proved to be very rewarding. By the time we had reached this stage of the treatment, Daisy was "on my side" and had accepted this "weird" approach. The first hold for unwinding was to place the hands on either side of the knee joint (with the knee supported and slightly flexed on a bean bag). The hands were in place for what seemed like ages (five minutes), while there was much internal twisting and turning in the joint itself. Since there was enough time left over left in our session, I decided to unwind between the knee and the lower lumbar spine, which proved quite easy to accomplish.   ·

5. I again mobilized the joint and put it through a full range passive movements—as I did with the other knee. Daisy got off the couch and took a few steps around the room. A huge beaming smile appeared on her face. This was the first time in months that she had been able to put full weight on her knee without being in excruciating pain. We agreed to meet again in one week.

Second Treatment Session

Daisy had been relatively pain-free for about two days before the pain had crept back again, but not as much as before. She reported, though, that she had had more backache. I had expected this. She did have quite bad osteoarthritis in the lumbosacral junction, the pain of which had been masked by the more acute pain in the knee. With the knee joint feeling a little better, the brain now picked up on the pain in the spine. She was more than happy to receive some more treatment. Although she was partly undressed in this session so that I could treat her lower spine, she commenced the treatment lying supine.

1. The first part of the treatment was much the same as the previous session, although there was more freeing up and mobilizing of the feet. Each stage was as before, but the energy balancing did not take as long.

2. After the knee treatment, Daisy turned over in to prone lying so that I could concentrate on the lower spine. This was massaged and mobilized, especially with CTM.

3. I stimulated the posterior Base chakra and then balanced it with the posterior Sacral chakra point. The X-rays that she had brought along showed that she had gross osteoarthritic changes in the L5-S1 facet joints, with some wear and tear around L4-5 as well. Since it was a large lesion area, I placed my whole hand over the area and balanced with the Base chakra point until a change of emphasis occurred.

4. The lesion was then balanced with both of the Knee chakras, the posterior Sacral chakra, and the upper cervical region.

5. I proceeded to unwind by placing one hand on the lesion area and the other over the upper cervical region. This was followed by placing both hands on either side of the spine at the lower lumbar area.

6. Finally, the lower lumbar region was mobilized further. Daisy arose from the couch and took a few steps. Following a great deal of initial stiffness (she was not been accustomed to lying on her front), she felt much easier in the knee and the lower spinal region. We agreed to meet in one week.

Third Treatment Session

Daisy had felt much better during the week; she even felt like doing some of the chores that had become difficult to do. Her sleeping pattern had become more regular, and she had felt better within herself (it is amazing how much better people feel without constant pain). With the maxim "don't change a winning formula" foremost in my mind, I decided to do exactly the same treatment as I had before, concentrating more on the lower spine than on the knee. Daisy now comes for "service" once every three months or so. She remains hooked on chakra therapy and has told all of her friends about it!

Thoracic Scoliosis with Arthritic Changes
History

Jack was a fifty-five-year-old radiographer and had been told by specialists that he had either been born with or had acquired a scoliosis at a very young age. He recalls that from an early, he has had pain and tension between the shoulder blades, which often affected his breathing, since it seemed to cause tension in the diaphragm/solar plexus region. Over the past few years he has also experienced some cervical restriction and discomfort, which had been diagnosed as cervical spondylosis, but it was the thoracic condition that needed to be treated. Jack's pain was worse when he stood and sat and better when he lay down. There seemed to be quite a pronounced sympathetic nerve system inflammation, since he often felt very hot, sweaty, and occasional "fainting" sensations. He suffered badly from indigestion and bloating. (The sympathetic nerve chain, which is part of the autonomic nervous system, lies alongside the transverse processes of the thoracic spine and may be affected by constant mechanical irritation of the scoliosis and arthritis in the thoracic area.)

Jack informed me that he is on constant medication for the pain and spasm, including diazepam (Valium) for the tension. He has tried many types of therapy, including acupuncture, physical therapy, and reflexology. He had ruled out surgery to straighten the spine, because it would be too dangerous. Jack had decided to use chakra acupressure and bodywork, since he had been referred by a patient who had also received this therapy.

First Treatment Session

1. I started the session by doing some massage with effleurage and deep kneading along the spine. The Bladder meridian was also massaged, as were the intercostals spaces and "rib lines." The main lesion appeared to be at T7-8. This was the most painful vertebra, and this level gives its sympathetic nerve supply to the diaphragm. I mobilized the thoracic spine by pushing gently on the spinous and transverse processes. Jack informed me that when he had received some physical therapy, this part of the treatment had helped him.

2. Since Jack's condition was long-standing, I stimulated the posterior Base chakra for approximately four minutes in order to create a reservoir of energy in the spine as a whole. This was followed by balancing the posterior Base chakra point with the posterior Throat chakra at C7-T1 (Gov 14). This balance took quite some time to achieve, which is hardly surprising due to the inordinate length of time that there had been a spinal imbalance. I now energy balanced the lesion at T7 with the Base chakra until a change of emphasis occurred. This started to release the diaphragmatic tension.

3. The lesion area of T7 was now energy balanced with the posterior Solar Plexus chakra point at T12-L1 and the tender point on the

axillary line under the seventh rib. There were no other reflected areas with which to balance, since T7 represents the center of the spine. Later I taught Jack the reflexes on the feet and hands so that he could self-treat.

4. I again mobilized the thoracic region. It appeared that there was a little more movement than there had been. Jack certainly noticed much less spinal and diaphragmatic tension. We agreed to meet in a week.

Second Treatment Session

Jack commented that he had slept "like a baby" for three nights following the first treatment. His bowel had been working "overtime," and he had had more energy (all good stuff). Once again, not wishing to change a winning formula, I repeated the first treatment. I noticed that there was more movement in the thoracic vertebral joints (before they were "solid") and that there was generally more "energy" in the spine as a whole. The various balancings took much less time.

Since there was so much time left in our session, I decided to concentrate on balancing energy *through* the lesion by balancing the Base chakra and the Throat chakra until a change of emphasis was attained. This provoked a profound reaction. Jack's breathing pattern changed from relaxed to agitated, and within a few seconds he was forced to sit up. Emotion was written all over his face. I gave him some tissues, and he cried for some time. This was an amazing emotional release that had probably stimulated and brought to the surface the true cause of the problem. It is only by working with the chakra system that the true cause of some conditions may be ascertained. When he had composed himself, Jack could not recall what emotions had surged through him, except for fear and the feeling of being "trapped." I asked him to ponder this and to let me know the next time we met, which would be in one week.

Third Treatment Session

Once again, Jack had slept soundly and had felt wonderfully relaxed. He had quizzed his mother during the week as well as others who knew him when he was a baby and child. His mother informed him that his had been a difficult birth and that he had been born with the cord around his neck. This experience had probably created a lot of inner tension, which had been expressed through diaphragmatic and solar plexus tension caused by his not breathing correctly for some minutes. It is possible that the scoliosis came about as a result of the deep muscle tension. Jack was confident that the cause of the problem had been addressed. The treatment was repeated, although this time there were no emotional outbursts. Jack came to see me regularly once a month or every six weeks to keep the thoracic spine "freed up" and for a general energy balance with acupressure or acupuncture. This case history reinforces the fact that it is more than possible for a therapist to seek out the deepest-seated of conditions and to find the true cause with bodywork.

Chronic Tennis Elbow
History

Beverly was a thirty-four-year-old company secretary who had suffered from pain in her left elbow for about two years. She had tried splint supports, bandages, magnets, acupuncture, and physical therapy and had received two cortisone injections. Each treatment had helped her a little, but the pain had returned soon after. Beverly also suffered from neck pain, headaches, light-headedness, and pins and needles in her thumb. My initial thoughts that it may be a dominant C5-6 lesion giving referred pain to the elbow were quashed when she informed me that she had also received some osteopathy that had concentrated on the neck and had made no difference at all.

Examination

Beverly appeared to be a very nervous woman (she may have been thinking that nothing was going to help). She was right-handed, so the problem was on the nondominant arm. There was obvious pain and discomfort over the origin of the extensor digitorum muscle of the left elbow. The lower cervical area was tense, but I concluded that it was not the cause of the problem, since there were no appreciable joint misalignment or nerve root signs to warrant it.

1. Beverly was comfortable lying supine with me sitting by her side. I began treatment with long massage strokes along the course of the meridians, followed by short strokes around the elbow. This elicited much discomfort. Mobilizing of the radioulnar joint proved to be very painful.

2. I stimulated the distal chakra point of the Hand chakra for a few minutes. This was followed by energy balancing between the Hand chakra and the Shoulder chakra in an attempt to create energy through the elbow joint. All this time, Beverly's arm was tense; so far nothing had seemed to help.

3. The lesion point was very easy to find. I energy balanced it with the Hand chakra until a change of emphasis occurred. This took a long time, but as soon as we reached the magical point, the tissues in the elbow appeared to be more relaxed and less painful. The lesion was then energy balanced with the knee on the same

side of the body and the other elbow. It was also balanced with the Shoulder chakra and posterior Throat chakra.

4. I concluded the treatment with some more deep massage and mobilizing. The elbow generally felt a little easier, but since she had "been there before," Beverly did not allow herself to get excited.

Second Treatment Session

Beverly reported that she had been blessed (her words) with some degree of comfort for the first time in a long while, but there was still a long way to go (again, her words).

First I administered massage and mobilizing as before, and neither appeared to be as painful as it had before.

The remainder of the treatment was the same. While I was energy balancing the lesion and the posterior Throat chakra (attempting to ease tension in the neck), Beverly started chatting about her work, her boss, and her general displeasure with both. Suddenly, bells were ringing that the real cause of the problem had now presented itself. In the school of body language, elbow conditions may be caused by the person's inability to get out of a rut and to "break free." It is generally the Throat chakra that is affected by a lack of self-expression, but experience in treating these lesions has taught me that if there is much overall tension in the cervicothoracic region, this may affect the nerve flow from the area and give a referred "tension." Coupled with this, the elbow is a "pivot" joint that may become affected when the person is uncertain about her future. I put this scenario to Beverly, and she admitted she had also thought about it She had been thinking about quitting her job for ages, but nothing else had come along. Fortuitously, she was going for an interview in two days. I spent the remainder of the treatment helping the "physical" tension at the neck and elbow. She promised to telephone me after the interview.

Beverly telephoned me a few days later to say that she had done well in the interview and had been offered the job. She had given a month's notice at her old job. She called me four weeks later to tell me that while she had been working her last weeks at the old job, her elbow had become unbearable. As soon as she had started working for the new company, the elbow had been the best it had been for months. Three months down the line, she is completely pain-free. Although the chakra acupressure therapy had merely highlighted the actual cause of her discomfort, no physical therapy could have achieved anything, since the true cause was an emotional one. Food for thought!

CHAPTER FOUR

Reflexology

This chapter is dedicated to the untold number of therapists who practice reflexology (or reflextherapy, as I prefer to call it). It will show how reflexology can be performed using the reflected chakra points on the feet and hands. I will also refer to the scores of other reflected points on the body.

To use the reflected chakras, you do not need a reflexology diploma, although the experienced gained from completing a diploma course will help. It is often sufficient just to have sensitive hands. Here I offer a brief history of reflexology for those readers who are unfamiliar with this therapy.

Foot reflexology has been around as long as acupuncture and acupressure and has its roots in Traditional Chinese Medicine. The modern practice of "zone therapy" began with an American ENT specialist, Dr. William Fitzgerald. He noticed that his patients varied in the amount of postoperative pain from which they suffered. Fitzgerald also discovered that those patients who had performed their own kind of "painful point therapy" on the feet fared better than those who were ignorant of such procedures. After researching this phenomenon he discovered that the human body can be divided into ten equal sections (five on each side of the body) along its vertical plane from head to feet. These sections were not just on the

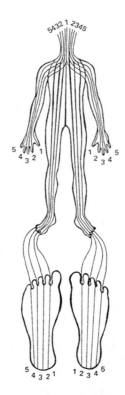

BODY & FEET ZONES

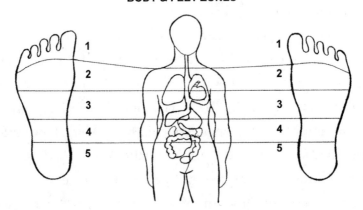

LEVEL OF REFLEXES ON THE FEET

FIGURE 4.1

Horizontal and Vertical Zones of the Body and Feet

skin but appeared to affect the underlying organs as well. An American masseuse, Eunice Ingham, interested in Dr. Fitzgerald's work, concentrated her efforts on mapping out both vertical and horizontal zones on the feet, as well as body points. She invented what is a major philosophy of reflexology, called foot zonal therapy. In the beginning, this therapy concentrated on the joints, mainly of the hands and feet, with the use of heavy pressure lasting up to a few minutes. This type of reflexology has since become the most popular form used in the West. Figure 4.1 shows the horizontal and vertical zones of the body, along with the levels of reflexes on the feet.

TYPES OF REFLEXOLOGY

Since the advent of the original foot zonal therapy, other forms of reflexology have emerged. Some of them encompass zone therapy, but others use the Chinese meridian system, the organic system, and the organic-joint system; some use a total energetic principle. Each of the types assumes that the whole of the body can be mapped on the feet, thus giving a microcosm within the macrocosm. Types of reflexology include "foot reflexology," "hand reflexology," "vertical reflextherapy," "organic reflexology," "universal reflexology," "zone therapy," and "light touch reflexology." There are several more concepts to consider. The amount of pressure that you use on your patient depends on the type of reflexology that you have studied and practiced. This ranges from using extremely heavy massage on tender points to hardly touching at all. Thus there appears to be a variety of ideas about and approaches to this wonderful form of healing.

Whatever type of reflexology you use, the rationale behind the treatment is to affect the many reflexes or reflected areas of the body by the use of touch or massage, to bring relaxation, harmony, and homoeostasis (energy balance) to the area. The effect of the treatment session may be felt immediately, soon afterward, the following day, or even two days later. Reflexes, of course, appear on many other areas of the body, apart from the feet. It is thought that there are as many as fourteen areas of reflexes (or reflected areas) on the body that can be used for diagnostic purposes and ten reflected areas that can be used for treatment.

The diagnostic areas are the iris, tongue, teeth, face, temple, pulse, hand, skull, ear, foot, abdomen, and spine as well as the meridians and the major and minor chakras. The areas that can be used for treatment are on the ear, skull, temple, face, hands, feet, abdomen, spine, meridians, and chakras. Although reflex points appear other places on the body, in this chapter we will concentrate on using the reflected chakras on the feet and hands. (For a full description of the other reflected pathways and areas on the body, please see my two previous books on acupressure and reflextherapy, as well as the chapter I wrote on "Naturopathy" in *Complementary Therapies for Physical Therapists*.)

Reflexology is a wonderful form of therapy that can have enormous impact on the patient suffering from both acute and chronic maladies. Although it is true that all types of reflexology are effective, it is also apparent that some are more effective than others. Before I came up with using the chakra approach on the hands and feet, the type of reflexology that seemed effective was the one using light touch and that recognized the fact that reflexes are meant to be gently massaged and not pulverized! I have lost track of the number of practitioners I have seen giving harsh treatments that rendered their patients speechless in agony or shouting in pain as they hovered several inches above the couch. There is never any need for harsh and deep reflexology. Reflexes become tender and sore if the associated body part is in a state of imbalance. This should be used as a signal from the patient that something is wrong, so the reflexes should be respected and not beaten into submission by heavy-handed massage.

I have always been an advocate of light touch reflexology, with an understanding that reflexology works via the energy system of the body (which in turn is governed by the central nervous system). Experience has shown that the lighter the touch, the more powerful the treatment and its effect. This, though, has to be coupled with the *inten-*

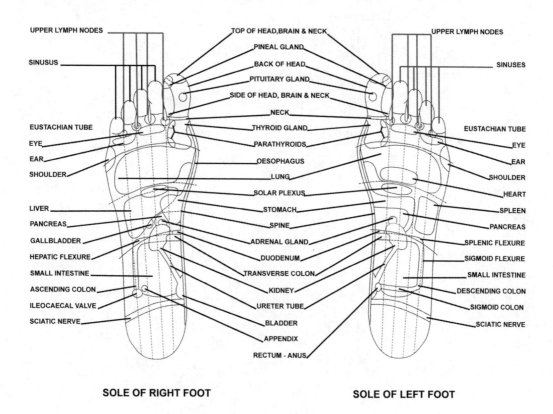

SOLE OF RIGHT FOOT   **SOLE OF LEFT FOOT**

FIGURE 4.2
Foot Reflexes in a Typical Foot Reflexology Chart

tion of the therapist. As with most touch therapies, reflexology always works best if the practitioner treats with empathy, love, and purpose. Figures 4.2 and 4.3 show typical reflexology foot and hand charts.

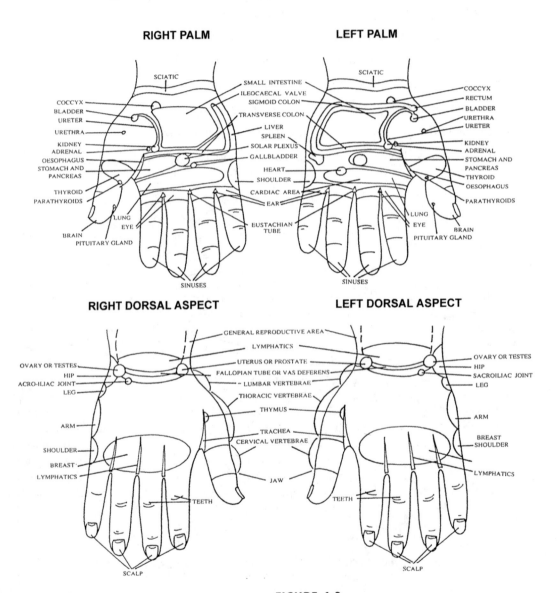

FIGURE 4.3

Hand Reflexes in a Typical Hand Reflexology Chart

THE REFLECTED CHAKRAS

The reflected aspects of the seven major chakras may be easily found on both the feet and the hands. As you would expect, their positioning mirrors their placement on the body. The lower five chakras are positioned along the medial aspects of the feet and hands. The Brow chakra is placed in the middle of the large toe and thumb to signal the positioning of the third eye and pituitary gland. The Crown chakra is positioned on the tips of the large toe and thumb. The twenty-one minor chakras are also positioned as one would expect them to be. Those minor centers that are located on the lateral aspect of the body, for example, the Ear, Intercostal, and Shoulder, are positioned on the lateral aspect of the foot and hand. Also found on the lateral aspect are those minor chakras found on the limbs, for example, the Knee, Elbow, Hand, and Foot. The Clavicular, Navel, and Groin chakras are positioned along the second zone—the Clavicular being on a horizontal line between the Shoulder and the Throat, the Navel being in between the Solar Plexus and the Sacral, and the Groin being just lateral to the Base. There is purposely no position for the Spleen chakra. The properties of this chakra are very similar to those of the Solar Plexus, Navel, and Sacral chakras, and it is superfluous to try to use it as well as the other three. Perfectionists may argue that it should be positioned where the spleen reflex is—on the fourth zone of the left foot, but please remember that the Spleen chakra is not the same as the spleen organ. In over twenty-eight years of practicing this therapy, I have never needed to use it.

Figures 4.4 and 4.5 show the reflected chakras on the feet and hands. Although using the exact positioning with the fingers on the point is desirable in achieving the desired effect, as with most acu-

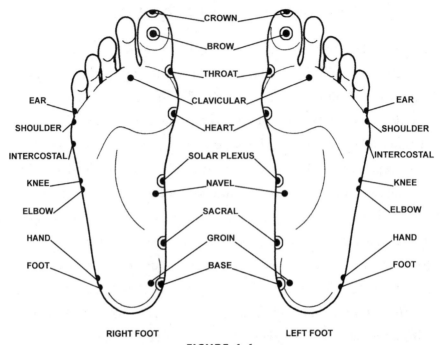

FIGURE 4.4

Reflected Major and Minor Chakras on the Feet

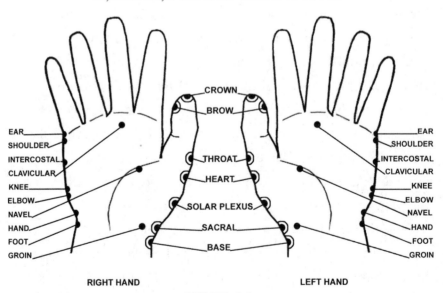

FIGURE 4.5

Reflected Major and Minor Chakras on the Hands

point and reflex points on the body, there is an area of influence around the point. Experience, however, will tell you when you are *on* or *nearly on* the point—there appears to be a difference to the touch compared with that on other reflex areas of the feet. This sensation is difficult to describe; all I can say is that it feels "magnetic." That is, once the fingers are placed on the reflected chakra points, they will be magnetically "held" in position for the duration of the particular balance or treatment. As described earlier, the body chakra points are very powerful and influence a kind of magnetic resonance around them; this occurs in a similar way on the chakra reflexes, though not as strongly. The major chakra points seem to be magnetically stronger than the minor ones. A technique of using the reflected chakras in the physical-etheric aura to make use of this extra magnetic power is described in the next chapter.

PRETREATMENT REGIMEN

It is very important to give patients sufficient time to "unwind" from the stresses and strains of their day or the journey to see you. Small talk *is* important in that it allows them time to relax. The patient should be comfortable and warm, either lying supine, long sitting on a couch, or seated comfortably on a purpose-built reflexology Relaxor.

The patient's feet should be exposed and at the correct comfortable height for you. It is imperative that you be just as comfortable as the patient. Next, the feet should be gently massaged. This should feel relaxing for the patient, but it also allows you to initially gauge the general demeanour of the feet (which, of course, mirrors the body as a whole). There is always debate about whether or not to use massage oil. Experience has shown that it helps in that it provides a friction-free surface on which to work. It will also help when treating patients with slightly sweaty feet. The massage should last a few minutes and should encompass the lower legs and all the toes. Some passive joint mobilizing should also be performed at this stage. Stiff joints are very common in all chronic disease. Patients adore foot mobilizing, with the rare exception of those who have sensitive feet.

INITIAL HOLDS

Following the opening massage, one of three initial holds should be carried out depending on the type of condition presented. These serve to initiate the energy balancing and are as follows:

- In cases of tension and anxiety, hold point KID 1.
- In all acute conditions, hold the toes.
- In all chronic cases, hold the heels.

The Use of Acupoint KID 1 (Kidney 1)

KI D1 is situated in the middle zone of the sole (plantar aspect) of the foot approximately two-thirds from the heel and one third from the tip of the middle toe. In reflexology it approximates with the upper and middle aspect of the diaphragm and is just proximal to the solar plexus reflex. It is the only acupoint on the sole of the foot and is usually called the Foot chakra point. It should be thought of as the initial contact point with the patient, following massage and mobilizing, in all cases of tension, stress, and anxiety, regardless of the overall picture presented by the patient. It can be a really magical point when used correctly. (See Figure 4.6.)

Begin by gently touching bilateral KID 1 with the pads of the middle fingers. After about two minutes of just touching the points (do not stimulate them), a change of emphasis should be felt. It will be at this moment that the patient will start to feel more relaxed. The point may be held for a further couple of minutes or so if you feel there is a need. KID 1 also answers well when treated in the etheric body—this will be discussed in the last chapter. If you find it difficult to place the fingers on the point for such a long time, try to rest your forearms on the end of the couch and cross your arms so that the right middle finger is touching the patient's right foot and left is on left. It is a much more comfortable position to hold. KID 1 is also used extensively with chakra healing in acupressure (sometimes acupuncture) and magnetic therapy. As stated in Chapter 2 it is associated with the Hand chakra and the Crown chakra. You may then proceed to holding the toes or heels, depending on whether or not the condition is acute or chronic. When using hand reflexology, the Hand chakra at point PC 8 is used. This is particularly useful when it is not convenient for the patient to take his or her shoes and socks off. It is also an excellent way of self -calming—try it, it really works! It represents a much better point than the highly used and misused LI 4 point.

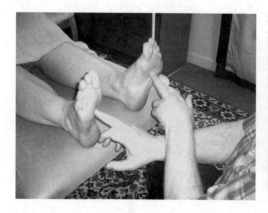 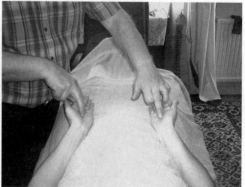

FIGURE 4.6a and 4.6b
Holding Point KID 1 and Holding Point PC 8

Acute Conditions: Holding the Toes

Acute conditions are those that appear to arrive quickly and usually disappear just as quickly with the correct treatment. They can range from a sore throat to an upset stomach. This section will usually just apply to the treatment of family and friends, since patients do not really consult therapists about such conditions.

The toes are the appendages of the feet and in TCM are considered to govern the acute or "yang" symptoms, whereas the heels govern chronic or "yin" symptoms. Your forearms must be supported with the hands placed totally over the patient's toes in a "wrapped-around" mode—see Figure 4.7. The action of holding the toes for a couple of minutes prior to the main thrust of the treatment serves two purposes. First it acts as a measure of or guide to the general yang condition of the patient. Second, it helps to bring the yang energies into homeostasis, thus allowing the patient's energies to relax. The sensation felt under the fingers is generally one of heat and tingling—often the hands appear to become red hot. While your hands are becoming warmer (through a combination of conduction, convection, and magnetic energy flow) the patient appears to be slightly cooler and more relaxed and settled. Holding the toes does *not* treat the specific complaint but allows general yang energy balancing to occur. Following toe holding, the treatment may proceed toward specific ailment therapy (described later) or to holding the heels as in the case of yang symptoms with an underlying yin cause.

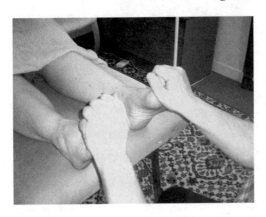

FIGURE 4.7
Holding the Toes

Chronic Conditions: Holding the Heels

Holding the heels represents a truly wonderful way of assessing, balancing, and treating the patient's energy system—basically by keeping the hands quite still. In my book *Acupressure and Reflextherapy in Medical Conditions*, I described using the vault hold of the skull and the heels as "listening posts." I have received enormous feedback on this topic, and the workshops on this topic have had to become longer just to accommodate this extra knowledge. Virtually every patient who consults you will have some form of chronic disease process, so the pre-treatment regimen discussed below is well worth learning, even though you may not be a practicing reflexologist.

Position

Make sure that the patient is comfortable and that your forearms are supported. You could be holding the heels for up to fifteen minutes, so it is imperative that you are comfortable. Both the heels should be "cuddled," that is, hold the left heel in the right hand, and the right heel in the left hand. (See Figure 4.8.)

General Energy Assessment

To assess the patient's general energy levels, the heels need to be held for at least a couple of minutes. Try not to move your hands (even slightly) or to adopt any mental intention. At the end of about two minutes, a certain amount of heat, tingling, or other sensation will be present. Generally speaking, if there

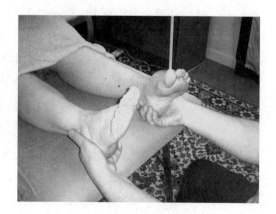

FIGURE 4.8
Holding the Heels

is a warm glow between you and your patient's heels, the energies are roughly balanced. In this case, specific treatment may be commenced. One heel may be warm, and the other may be cool or sticky—this shows energy imbalance, and you should proceed to using the heels in balancing mode. If there is very little warmth or glow of any kind under the heels, this indicates an extreme yin situation, and you should proceed to energy balancing mode. When the heels are occasionally sticky and damp, this indicates a great lack of vital force within the internal organs.

Balancing the Patient's General Energy

The heels represent a wonderful vehicle through which the patient's general energy may be balanced. Please note that in chronic illness the balance will not occur in just one treatment session; it may take three or even four. For this and the following techniques, it is essential that you "tune in" to the patient's energy flow. This is very similar to the energy tuning that is done in craniosacral therapy or cranial osteopathy using the vault hold. Craniosacral therapy purists insist that it is the rhythm or flow of the cerebrospinal fluid that is felt when one is using the vault hold. As mentioned in my first book, one's training guides one's philosophies on the subject. It is obvious that the cerebrospinal fluid motion cannot be felt in the heels, but it is also obvious that the patient's vital force (chi) as transmitted by the general fluid structure of the body in blood, lymph, and synovial fluid *can* be detected. The heels should be held for at least two minutes, and a slight change of emphasis must be felt. Once this has occurred, try to pick up the chi flow within the body; you can do this by sensing a gentle expansion and contraction under the heels.

When you have felt this, try to expand this sensation under the

hands to create a "balloon" effect of energy. This inward and outward motion that has been created is exactly the same as tuning into
the cerebrospinal fluid flow at the cranial base. An energy balance
has occurred when the same sensation exists under each heel and
the balloon effect is the same. For purposes of balancing energy try
to use the process of intention. In other words, visualize the expansion and contraction of energy in the heels. At the same time, you
may also move gently with the newfound rhythm.

Specific Analysis

To use this technique in analyzing individual organic energy imbalance, ask questions of the patient's energy system, as you would if
you were working with the vault hold at the cranial base. Once a
regular chi rhythm is felt, try asking specific questions regarding the
state of the individual chakras or internal organs. Each of the silently
asked questions must have a "yes" or "no" answer. For example,
you may silently ask if the Throat chakra needs treatment or if there
is sufficient energy flow within the spleen. When the answers to the
questions are negative, the flow remains; when the answer is positive,
the flow ceases. Questions can be tuned finer and finer until you
come to an exact diagnosis or analysis that will then help you to formulate the treatment. Remember it is the *positive* replies that change
the flow. This is the wonderful way in which the patient's energy
system is communicating with you in an attempt to show where the
cause of the imbalance lies. It is just one aspect of "body dowsing"—
more on this in the next chapter.

The Heels in Treatment Mode

There is no reason why treatment may not be done through the heels,

or at least initiated there. The feedback from many workshop delegates who have learnt this technique from me seems to suggest that
reflexologists really appreciate this extra dimension to their work.
There has to be a certain amount of mental "tuning in" to what is
being attempted. Since this takes time and patience, you may want
to cease small talk to allow greater concentration and intention to
occur. This is frequently no problem, since by the time you reach this
stage of the procedure, the patient is often too relaxed to want to talk
and in fact often falls asleep.

Make sure the expansion and contractions of the chi rhythm under
the heels are discernible, and proceed with the intention toward the
chakra or organ that you have decided is in need of treatment. For
instance, if the Throat chakra is sluggish, then this area needs total
concentration. It is hopeless in the extreme to think that this form of
energy therapy may be achieved successfully without total commit-
ment and concentration. Thoughts must *not* stray—it *has* to be 100
percent concentration.

Imagine that chi (healing) energy is travelling from the heels
toward the Throat chakra, for example, by mentally pushing it up
from the heels, up the legs and torso, and on to the throat area. While
you are doing this, the expansion and contraction flow of chi will be
lost—after all, this mode reflects balance and homoeostasis. This
may last for up to four to five minutes, during which time your concentration must not be lost. As soon as the patient exhibits signs of
change, for example, yawning, sighing, and so on, this will signal
that it is time once again to energy balance and that the treatment
has been successful. It is at this time that the expansion and contraction phase will once again be felt under the heels.

Many reflexologists are content to treat *just* through the heels and do not bother to carry out the specific treatment regimens detailed later. This is purely a personal thing—it does not mean that the treatment is any less effective or powerful.

GENERAL ENERGY BALANCING THROUGH THE REFLECTED CHAKRAS

Chapter 3 suggested that, on some occasions, balancing the energy of the chakras should be done prior to treatment of the individual chakra. There is no difference in reflexology. Balancing the reflected chakras serves to relax the patient, thus allowing the treatment phase to be carried out more easily. It also serves to highlight where the imbalance lies and which chakra(s) needs to be treated. Energy balancing with the reflected chakras is done in two phases—balancing left foot with right foot, and balancing top to bottom. Very light touch is used, and it is imperative to use the same fingers so as to obtain a magnetic balance. The middle fingers are the most popular, but it is perfectly all right to use the index fingers. The fingers are held in place until a similar sensation is felt underneath each finger. Experience has shown that it is more comfortable to cross the hands and to place the right finger on the patient's right foot and the left finger on the left foot. This holds good for the lower five chakras. When you reach the Brow chakra, it may be easier to uncross the hands.

Balancing Right Foot with Left Foot

The patient should be comfortable, and you should be able to place your forearms on the end of the couch so that they are well supported. Using the middle fingers pads and applying very gentle pressure, place the fingers on each of the Base chakra points situated at the lower end of the medial aspect of the heel. In every chronic disease, the Base chakra points are very sluggish, so it may be some time before balancing occurs. It is permissible to gently stimulate the points for a few seconds so as bring them "to life" before just holding them again. The balance should take no more than two to three minutes to achieve. It is not necessary to prolong the touch following balance, but it can be done if it feels like the right thing to do. This is especially appropriate if the chakras being balanced are the ones that eventually need treatment. There is no need to feel a true "change of emphasis" before proceeding to the next balance. Next move both middle fingers to the Sacral chakra at the level of the lower lumbar spine, and repeat the procedure. Then move them to the Solar Plexus, Heart, Throat, Brow, and Crown in that order. You will find that the sensation under the fingers and the texture of the feet will feel different the nearer to the toes the balancing is done. The balancing will not take as much time as the balancing of the "upper" chakras did.

Balancing Top to Bottom

Having balanced one foot with the other, it is now time to balance the chakra "couples." They are, in order, Heart with Solar Plexus; Throat with Sacral; Brow with Base; and Crown with Base. Please note that the Base chakra has the two couples of Brow and Crown, as it does with body chakra balancing. The technique is exactly the same as with balancing left and right feet. The middle two balances should be achieved fairly quickly, whereas the outer balancing involving the Base chakra will take a little longer, maybe two to three minutes. During the whole process of chakra balancing on the feet, you will become aware of the individual chakras that exhibit tendencies different from the norm. These differences may take the form of tardy balancing, different texture on the skin, local perspiration, and so on. The differences usually indicate that the particular chakra needs treatment (see the next section). The main point that I am making about balancing the reflected chakras is that although this process should not be rushed, it is still secondary in importance to the main treatment of the individual chakra. Having said that, it remains a powerful healing tool, and anything that brings about energy balancing and relaxation has to be good for the patient.

TREATMENT USING THE INDIVIDUAL REFLECTED CHAKRAS

Acute Conditions

This technique may be used to alleviate any acute, painful, or inflamed area of the body as well as treating subacute conditions and the acute, painful aspects of chronic conditions. There is undoubtedly a "painful" aspect to most chronic conditions, and it would be useful to use this technique in the early treatment stages of these conditions.

Principles of Treatment

The technique is simplicity itself. Place the middle finger of one hand on the most acute area of the reflected organ, that is, the exact reflected point of the acute condition. This could be an internal organ, joint, or muscular area—it doesn't matter. The middle finger of the other hand is then placed on the associated major chakra. The two fingers are held with very light touch with no massage or movement of any kind for about three or four minutes, or until there is a change in the pain or inflammation. The patient usually informs you that this has occurred, although at the very instance of a change of emphasis under the fingers he or she will tell you that the pain is easing. This remains a wonderful example of working *with* the patient and not doing something *to* them. I chose the following examples to include each of the major chakras. Also see Figure 4.9.

- *Pain in the right eye.* Hold the left middle finger on the eye reflex. There are several interpretations of this—choose the one that you have been taught or are comfortable with. Figure 4.9 shows the classical one on the heads of the metatarsals. Place the right middle finger on the Crown chakra reflex on the tip of the left big toe.

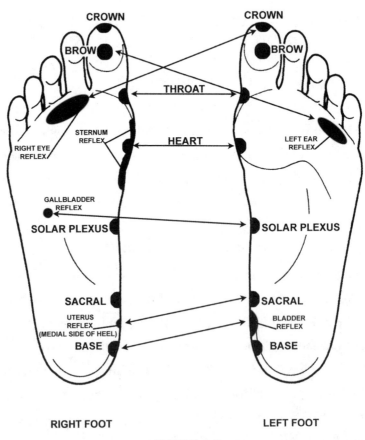

FIGURE 4.9

Using the Reflected Chakras in Acute Conditions

- *Pain in the left ear.* Hold the left middle finger on the reflected Brow chakra and the right middle finger on the left ear reflex. Once again, this may be found on the side of the big toe or at the head of the metatarsals.

- *Sore throat.* Hold one middle finger on the throat reflex on either foot and the other middle finger on the Throat chakra reflex. Since these two points are usually the same, the throat reflex is to be held on the foot that is on the pain side.

- *Midsternal or midthoracic pain.* Hold one middle finger on the painful reflex point on the sternum/thoracic area and the other middle finger on the Heart chakra reflex.

- *Gallbladder colic pain.* Hold the left middle finger on the gallbladder reflex and the right middle finger on the Solar Plexus chakra reflex on the left foot.

- *Menstrual pain.* Hold one middle finger on the most painful reflex point (this could be on the medial aspect of the foot) and the other middle finger on the Sacral chakra reflex.

- *Cystitis.* Hold one middle finger on the bladder reflex and the other middle finger on the Base chakra reflex of the opposite foot. Please try these holds—they really work!

Chronic Conditions

By their very nature, chronic conditions generally need much more time, patience and expertise to treat than acute ones. The reflexologist is generally used to spending several sessions in easing a chronic condition, so this is no different. It will be found, however, that fewer treatment sessions will be required when using this method. It doesn't always help the bank balance but the satisfaction of both practitioner and patient will make up for that.

Order of Treatment

1. Balance the reflected major chakra points foot to foot and top to bottom, as described earlier. It is imperative to balance at the beginning of every treatment. It does not matter if it is treatment session one or ten. You will find that as the condition improves and the vital force of your patient grows stronger, the balancing part of the session will become easier. Do not attempt to go beyond the point when the energy balance has been achieved, although it is tempting to do so.

2. Balance the associated major chakra reflex with the organ reflex. This procedure represents the main thrust of the treatment and as such should take some time. It takes into account the relationship between the individual chakra to be treated and its corresponding organs. The associated organs will mostly be in a yin state and therefore will need to be slightly stimulated. It also uses a more traditional reflexology approach that will enable you to use skills with which you may be more familiar.

   There are two phases to this section: (a) Stimulate/massage the associated reflex areas. These areas need to be massaged for up to half a minute, or longer if need be. If the area is desperate for treatment, it will feel congested and lacking in "fiber" and will need quite a lot of massage using the thumbs and forefingers. As stated before, it is not a question of digging the fingers in until the patient screams, but to perform fairly gentle and yet thorough massage. This should be done until you perceive definite tissue changes, that is, the tissues should feel more elastic, warmer, and generally more "energized"—any competent reflexologist will know exactly what is meant by this. (b) Balance a focal point of the associated reflex with the reflected major chakra. The focal point of the reflex is the point or points that exhibit the most tenderness when the reflex is massaged. This tender point is usually the "symptomatic" point, that is, the one point on the reflected area that best reflects the most symptomatic area in the body. In the case of a large reflected area, there may be more than one symptomatic point. Each must be balanced and treated separately.

It is important to state here that not all seven of the reflected chakras need to be treated. You only need to treat the ones presenting symptoms. You will know which ones need treatment from the knowledge of the condition that you have gleaned from the patient or because of the failure to balance the reflected chakra during the balancing phase. Once the focal (symptomatic) point is found, it needs to be balanced with the associated reflected chakra. When these two points are close together (as they often are), it is perfectly acceptable and even desirable to balance with the chakra point on the other foot. It is doubtful that an energy balance will be achieved quickly—there would be no point in treating the chakra if that were the case! Therefore the two points will probably need to be initially stimulated. This may take over a minute to do until the tissues start to relax a little. When you feel that they have, hold the two points, maybe for a further two or three minutes, until a change of energy emphasis is achieved (see Chapter 3). As soon as the change of emphasis has occurred and both parties are at the A/T state of consciousness, the tissues will feel very warm, comfortable, and pliable. There is almost a "warm putty" sensation. It is a good thing to keep this hold for longer than necessary. This is the crux of the treatment, and the longer the two points are held, the better will be the result.

3. Balance the associated reflected major chakra with its minor chakra

couple. Now that the focal point has been balanced with the major chakra, this needs to be reinforced with other components of the chakra complex. It is now that the reflected major chakra is balanced with the minor chakra couples. This is in contrast to the acupressure routine where the actual lesion is energy balanced with the chakra. When it is the reflex of the area that is being addressed (as in this chapter), the important thing to treat is the chakra—not the focal point. The latter merely represents the symptomatic point, whereas the chakra represents the cause. Each of the reflected major chakras has two associated minor chakras. The exceptions are the Solar Plexus and the Sacral, which "share" the reflected Spleen chakra. As with the previous part of the treatment, these two points may need to be stimulated at first in order to build up some energy to the area, before the two points can be energy balanced. Each one is done separately. The major chakra is balanced with one of the minor chakras, followed by a balance with the other one. If the condition warrants it, the two minor chakras may be balanced with each other. This is often a nice thing to do but not essential.

4. Balance the reflected chakra with the reflected Base chakra. This final part of the treatment procedure reinforces what has been achieved up to now. By energy balancing the reflected chakra with the Base chakra, you are creating a substantial foundation that will prevent the treatment from going "off the shelf" early. I often hear patients say that, following a session, they were much improved for a couple of days before their symptoms started to reappear. When the reflected chakra is supported with the Base chakra, this phenomenon does not usually occur. Naturally, when the affected reflected chakra is the Base chakra, this stage of the treatment need not be carried out.

In the next section, we will explore treatments of the individual chakras. See Figures 4.10 to 4.16.

TREATING INDIVIDUAL CHAKRAS
Crown Chakra

(See Figure 4.10.)

- The associated body systems are the upper brain (higher centers) and the right eye.
- The associated major chakra is the Base chakra.
- The associated minor chakras are the Hand and Foot chakras.
- The Endocrine gland is the Pineal.
- Possible symptoms are vertigo, high and low blood pressure, right-sided migraine, delusion, melancholy, and phobic tendencies.
- The reflected areas include the head (big toe) and the right eye reflex situated on the metatarsal heads underneath the second and middle toes of the right foot.

Order of Treatment

1. The first phase of the treatment is to balance the reflected chakras left to right and top to bottom as described previously.
2. The second phase is to gently massage the reflected area with thumb or finger pad, kneading until the tissues feel more relaxed. Make a note of the individual tender point(s) within the reflected area; this will be important later on. Take time in doing this, especially around the big toe with all its individual reflected parts.
3. The third phase is to balance the Crown chakra to the focal point of the reflected area. If a condition is affecting the head, for example, headaches, anxiety, or right-eye symptoms, the focal point

will relate to one of these areas. If the top of the head is exhibiting more symptoms, this should be held; if the right eye is giving more symptoms, then this point should be held. When balancing the focal point with the reflected Crown chakra, it is essential that this is done with one finger on the focal point and the other on the Crown chakra on the opposite foot—otherwise there is very little space between the points. Remember that in this phase a change of energy emphasis is to be reached. This is critical to the success of the treatment. Please remember to just "let it happen."

4. The next phase is to energy balance between the reflected Crown chakra and the reflected Foot chakra (not *the* Foot chakra at KID 1). This may be done on the same foot or the opposite foot; it does

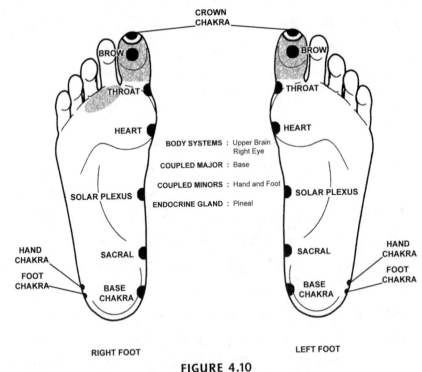

FIGURE 4.10

Crown Chakra Treatment

not matter. Now balance the reflected Crown chakra with the reflected Hand chakra. These two holds should not take too long

5. The final phase is to balance the reflected Crown chakra with the reflected Base chakra. This supports and reinforces the rest of the session, and it should take a couple of minutes before a change of emphasis is achieved. The patient will be feeling very relaxed by this stage. It essential to advise her to rest as much as possible during the day. Also tell her to drink plenty of water and not to eat anything too starchy or sugary.

Brow Chakra

(See Figure 4.11.)

- The associated body systems are the central nervous system, ears, nose, and left eye.
- The associated major chakra is the Base chakra.
- The associated minor chakras are the Clavicular and the Groin chakras.
- The endocrine gland is the pituitary.
- Possible symptoms are migraine; chronic catarrh; sinusitis; infectious and contagious disease; deafness and altered hearing; cervical spondylosis; Ménière' disease stress and worry-related symptoms; vertigo; dizziness; and brain "fog."
- Reflected areas include the big toes, the tips of all the toes (sinus reflexes), the ears, and the left eye (classical position beneath the toes).

Order of Treatment

1. The first phase of the treatment session is to balance the reflected major chakras left to right, and top to bottom as previously described.

2. Next, massage gently around the reflected areas. Take time doing this and try to ascertain "tender" (focal) points for use later on.

3. The next stage is to energy balance the reflected Brow chakra with the focal point previously deduced. This is the main thrust of the treatment session, and a change of emphasis must be achieved before proceeding to the next phase. Using points on opposite feet will be more comfortable for both practitioner and patient.

4. Now energy balance between the reflected Brow and the reflected Clavicular chakra, followed by balancing the Brow and the Groin chakras. It does not matter which foot is used, and it is not necessary to balance the two minor centers with each other.

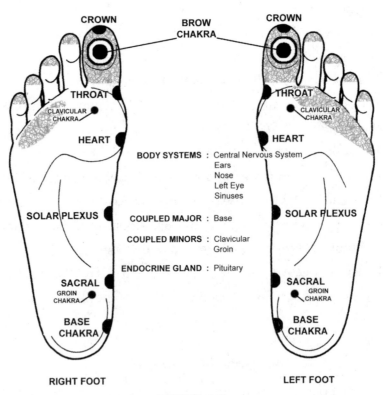

FIGURE 4.11
Brow Chakra Treatment

5. The final phase is to energy balance the reflected Brow center with the reflected Base chakra. This reinforces and supports the rest of the treatment, and care should be taken to attain a change of emphasis. Leave the patient with advice about relaxing, drinking lots of water, and not eating too much during the day. Also, teach him/her how to massage the reflected Brow chakra point on the thumbs (pituitary point), since this will augment the treatment. Make sure this point is massaged regularly; he/she will benefit from it.

Throat Chakra

(See Figure 4.12.)

- The associated body systems are the lungs, bronchi, vocal apparatus, alimentary canal, and upper limbs.
- The associated major chakra is the Sacral chakra.
- The associated minor chakras are the Shoulder and Navel chakras.
- The endocrine gland is the thyroid.
- Possible symptoms include migraine; chronic and acute sore throats; tonsillitis; asthma; shyness and introversion; loss of taste; chronic and acute bronchitis; colitis and irritable bowel syndrome; ileocaecal valve syndrome; and chronic skin lesions such as eczema and alopecia.
- Reflected areas include the lung areas and the large bowel areas on both feet.

Order of Treatment

1. The first phase is to energy balance the reflected chakras, left foot with right foot and top to bottom, as previously described
2. Second, massage the reflected areas on the soles of both feet. The area over the lungs should not be massaged with as much vigor

as the large bowel area. This is because of the delicate nature of the organ. Take care to ascertain the focal points that will be used later on. It could be that there may be two focal points, one related to respiratory system and one to the large bowel. It all depends on the overriding symptomatology of the patient.

3. Third, energy balance between the reflected Throat chakra and the focal point. Please be prepared to balance with the chakra on the opposite foot if the points are in close proximity. This is the pivotal part of the treatment, and a change of emphasis must be attained before proceeding to the next section.

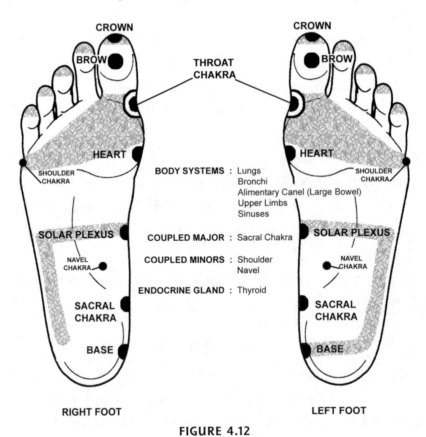

FIGURE 4.12
Throat Chakra Treatment

4. The reflected Throat chakra is now energy balanced with the reflected Navel chakra followed by balancing the reflected Throat chakra and reflected Shoulder chakra. The two minor chakras need not be balanced with each other.

5. Finally, energy balance the reflected Throat chakra with the reflected Base chakra so as to support and reinforce what has been achieved so far. A change of emphasis should be aimed for here, although in severely chronic cases of, say, chronic bronchitis, a balance may not be achievable in the first couple of treatments.

Since the Throat chakra is concerned with excretion (physical and emotional), please be prepared for two things that could occur during and after treatment. First, the patient may become very emotional as the deep seated emotional cause of the condition that has caused congestion in the Throat chakra is clearing—have tissues handy. Second, she must be warned that she may undergo some internal cleansing following the treatment session. This could be in the form of looseness of the bowel, skin eruption, oily skin, worsening of an existing skin condition, sinusitis, catarrh, or coldlike symptoms. Reassured the patient that all this is a perfectly normal naturopathic reaction and represents a huge stage in promoting homoeostasis within them.

Heart Chakra

(See Figure 4.13.)

- The associated body systems are the heart, circulation, and the vagus nerve.
- The associated major chakra is the Solar Plexus chakra.
- The associated minor chakras are the Ear and Intercostal chakras.
- The endocrine gland is the thymus.

- Possible symptoms include benign tumors and growths; cysts; heart conditions, ranging from heart failure to mitral stenosis; nausea; palpitations and tachycardia; varicosities; tearfulness; anxiety; vertigo; introversion; and shingles.
- Reflected areas include cover the heart region and the small intestine.

Order of Treatment

1. The first part of the treatment is to balance the reflected chakras left to right and top to bottom, as previously described.
2. The reflected areas around the heart and small intestine regions on

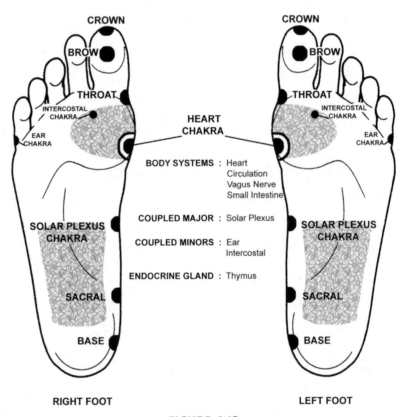

FIGURE 4.13

Heart Chakra Treatment

both feet should now be massaged, with care being taken to locate the focal points that could be used later on.

3. The reflected Heart chakra is now energy balanced with the focal point. This is the most important phase of the treatment and one that should be undertaken with due care and consideration. A change of emphasis should be achieved here before proceeding to the next phase. As with the previous example of the Throat chakra, when treating the Heart chakra, have tissues handy. Of all the chakras, imbalance in the Heart chakra is most often caused by emotional turmoil in the past. As with any form of naturo-pathic treatment, when the *cause* of the condition is addressed, the patient often reacts by "letting go" of that which caused the condition in the first place. He or she must be reassured that this is perfectly normal.

4. The reflected Heart chakra is now energy balanced with both the reflected Ear and the Intercostal chakras separately. There is no need to balance the two minor chakras with each other except in the case of shingles. Experience has shown that this balance helps to reinforce the treatment.

5. Finally, energy balance the reflected Heart chakra with the reflected Base chakra so as to support and reinforce what has already been achieved. A change of emphasis should be attained here. Advise the patient, as outlined above.

Solar Plexus Chakra

(See Figure 4.14.)

- The associated body systems are the stomach, liver, gallbladder, spleen, lymphatic circulation, and immune system.
- The associated major chakra is the Heart chakra.

- The associated minor chakra is the Spleen (and Sacral).
- The endocrine gland is the pancreas.
- Possible symptoms include skin conditions such as acne and eczema; stomach ulcers; cancerous growths; gallbladder colic; glandular fever; autoimmune system infection; allergies of *any* kind; chronic fatigue syndrome; hay fever; worry and depression; and anxiety.
- Reflected areas include the middle of the foot, plus the area on the dorsum of the foot associated with lymphatic drainage.

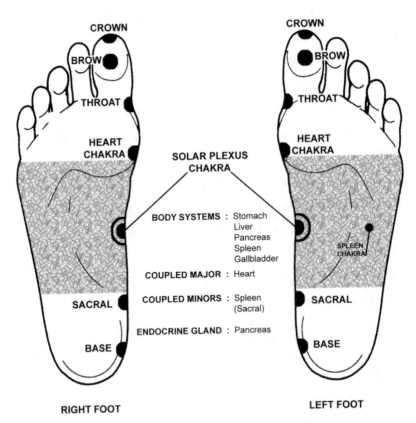

FIGURE 4.14

Solar Plexus Chakra Treatment

Order of Treatment

1. The first part of the treatment consists of balancing the reflected major chakras left to right and top to bottom.

2. Second, massage the reflected area. Remember to include the lymphatic area on the dorsum of the foot. Take care that you ascertain the focal point, since this information will be used later.

3. Now, energy balance the reflected Solar Plexus chakra with the focal point already highlighted. This is the pivotal part of the treatment, and care should be taken that the correct points are being used. A change of emphasis should be attained before proceeding to the next phase.

4. The next phase is to energy balance the reflected Solar Plexus chakra with the reflected Spleen chakra. Please note that there is only one reflected Spleen chakra point on the left foot. When the patient is suffering from any immune deficiency condition such as chronic fatigue syndrome, glandular fever, or *any* allergy, the reflected Solar Plexus should also be balanced with the reflected Sacral chakra. It also helps if the two "minor" chakras are balanced with each other. The Solar Plexus, Sacral, and Spleen chakras represent the triad of chakras that are involved with all these conditions. When treating a patient who has cancer, these three chakras also need to be used. This is imperative. Please remember that no one who is working in the complementary medicine field or who is a nonregistered medical practitioner can state that they are treating cancer (as well as diabetes and venereal disease). There is, however, no reason why a cancer patient cannot consult you. Their vital force could be enhanced tremendously so that their bodies can endure the conventional (and sometimes caustic) medical procedures that are targeting the cancer.

5. The final phase is to energy balance the reflected Solar Plexus chakra with the reflected Base chakra. This supports and reinforces the treatment already carried out. Give suitable advice about resting adequately and drinking plenty of water for the next twenty-four hours.

Sacral Chakra

(See Figure 4.15.)

- The associated body systems are the reproductive system, the lymphatic circulation, and fluid balance.
- The associated major chakra is the Throat chakra.
- The Associated minor chakra is the Spleen (and the Solar Plexus) chakra.
- The associated endocrine gland is the gonads or uterus.
- Possible symptoms are low vitality; chronic tiredness and fatigue; impotence; high or low libido; sore throats; edema; imbalance with "heating mechanism," including chilblains and cold extremities; menstrual and menopausal symptoms; and some rheumatoid conditions.
- Reflected areas lie along the medial, underside, and lateral aspects of the heels. Added to this area are the lymphatic areas (as per Solar Plexus chakra) and the areas on the medial and lateral aspects of the feet that are associated with the reproductive organs.

Order of Treatment

1. The first part of the treatment is to energy balance the reflected chakras left to right and top to bottom, as previously described.
2. Second, massage all the reflected areas associated with the Sacral chakra. Take care to include them all and to make note of the

point(s) that are most tender. With Sacral chakra imbalance there is invariably more than one focal point. The reason is that when there is a congested Sacral chakra, this gives rise to chronic and long-standing conditions that could produce many other disease factors. The other point to consider is that the patient is often extremely tired, owing to their various vital force imbalances. The tissues will appear sluggish and lacking in vitality, so please proceed with caution. It does *not* mean that you should adopt a gung-ho attitude by overstimulating all the reflected areas. The reverse is true. The reflected areas should be massaged with a feather-

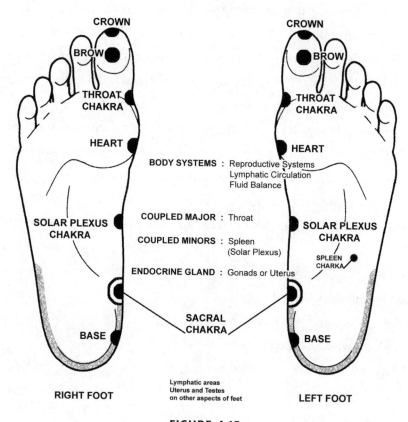

FIGURE 4.15

Sacral Chakra Treatment

light touch. Always remember that the subtler the approach, the more powerful will be the treatment and the less likely it will be for any "treatment trauma" and adverse reaction to crop up. This cannot be stated too strongly.

3. Third, energy balance the reflected Sacral chakra point with the focal point(s) already found. This has do be done with great care, since it is the most important part of the procedure. A change in energy emphasis has to be attained here before proceeding to the next phase. With two or more points of focus, they have to be balanced separately. This does take time, but keep in mind that the whole session lasts no longer than a more conventional reflexology treatment.

4. The reflected Sacral chakra is now balanced with the reflected Spleen and Solar Plexus chakras, as described in the previous section. Balance the three as in a triad.

5. Finally, energy balance the reflected Sacral chakra with the reflected Base chakra. This is to support and reinforce what has been achieved so far. The patient must be warned that he may feel very tired and to just "go with the flow" and not to fight it. he must also drink a lot of clear tap water.

Base Chakra

(See Figure 4.16.)

- The associated body systems are the spinal column, lower limbs, kidneys, bladder, and skeletal system.
- The associated major chakras are the Crown and Brow chakras.
- The associated minor chakras are the Elbow and Knee chakras.
- The associated endocrine gland are the adrenals.
- Possible symptoms include osteoarthritis; ankylosing spondyli-

tis; cervical spondylosis; thoracic scoliosis and arthritis; stiff joints; peripheral joint arthritis; lethargy and chronic fatigue; chronic cystitis and nephritis; prostatitis; gravitational ulcers; Scheurmann's disease and other bone-related conditions; depression; and low spirits.

- Reflected areas include the medial aspect of the foot (spinal reflex), the lateral aspect of the foot and the kidney, and the urethra and bladder areas.

Order of Treatment

1. The first phase of the treatment is to energy balance the reflected chakras left to right and top to bottom, as previously described.

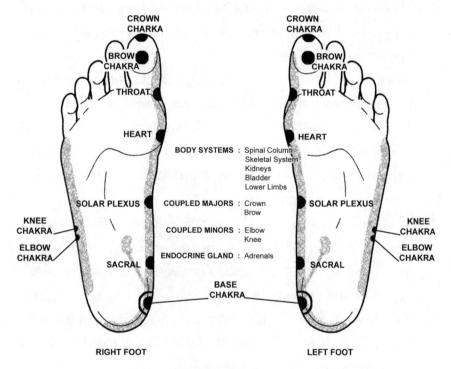

FIGURE 4.16
Base Chakra Treatment

2. Second, massage the medial and lateral aspects of the feet, plus the kidney and bladder areas. Take care to notice the focal point, since this will be needed later in the treatment. With all Base chakra imbalances, there is chronic sluggishness of the tissues. The same advice holds true with the treatment of the Sacral chakra imbalance—do not use heavy-handed massage! The philosophy of "subtle is powerful" can be difficult to understand, especially when the reflexologist is used to using heavy massage with chronic conditions. A leap of faith is often required to accept this new paradigm. Once learnt and practiced, it is never forgotten.

3. Now it is time to energy balance the focal point (s) with the reflected Base chakra. This is the most important part of the treatment session, and care should be taken that the correct points are being used. A change of emphasis should always be attained here, if possible.

4. Now energy balance the reflected Base chakra with its associated minor chakras, the reflected Elbow and Knee chakras. Try for a change in emphasis if the knee or elbow is the main condition. There is no need to balance the reflected Knee and Elbow chakras with each other unless there are arthritic changes in both joints (a very rare circumstance).

5. Finally, instead of energy balancing with the reflected Base chakra as is done with all the others, balance the reflected Base chakras on the left and right foot with each other. Although you carried this out in the first phase of the treatment, when you have this part of the session, you will feel quite a change compared to earlier on. Try for a change of emphasis. Follow up the treatment with advice to the patient about resting and drinking plenty of water.

CASE HISTORIES OF USING CHAKRA REFLEXOLOGY

We conclude this chapter with some more case histories of my patients.

Irritable Bowel Syndrome

This condition is very common and answers very well to this approach.

History

Diane, age fifty-two, had been suffering from IBS for about fifteen years. She also has had mild eczema on her arms and legs, catarrh, occasional painful sinusitis, headaches when concentrating or reading, sore throats, painful knees, and varicose veins. Diane had also suffered through menopause, which was now (mercifully) over. She had tried taking dairy produce out of her diet with little or no affect.

Given these symptoms, I decided that probably the Throat and Sacral chakras needed to be treated, but this would be reinforced when energy balancing.

First Treatment Session

1. I massaged the feet and lower legs with a little oil, taking care not to massage over the varicose regions. Some edema was present, and the general feeling of the tissues was sluggish, indicating poor lymphatic drainage.
2. The reflected chakras were energy balanced left to right feet and top to bottom. I noted that both the reflected Base, Sacral, and Throat chakras were congested and did not want to energy bal-

ance with their coupled chakras. I decided to treat the reflected Sacral chakra, followed by the reflected Throat chakra.

3. Since there was only time to treat one of them today, I chose the Sacral chakra. I gently massaged the reflected areas of the Sacral chakra, including the lymphatic and sexual areas. A focal point was found (not surprisingly) on the uterus point.

4. This point was then energy balanced with the reflected Sacral chakra, which took quite some time to bring about, reflecting the chronicity of the condition.

5. Finally, the reflected Sacral chakra was balanced with the reflected Base chakra. I advised Diane to drink lots of tap water and to exercise in moderation.

Second Treatment Session

Diane came back to see me a week later. She had been very tired and had slept much better than usual. In the past few days had had a little more energy than before. Her throat had been very sore, and she had been doing some aspirin gargles. I decided to treat the Throat chakra.

1. The feet and lower legs were massaged, with the tissues feeling more pliable and "energized" than before.

2. The reflected chakras were balanced left to right and top to bottom. Once again it was the Throat and Sacral chakras that did not balance.

3. The reflected areas of the Throat chakra were massaged—lungs, bronchi, alimentary canal and throat regions. I also decided to massage the Sacral chakra regions again. The focal point on the Throat chakra areas was the throat region, which was very tender.

4. I balanced this tender point with the reflected Throat chakra on

the opposite foot. It seemed to take an eternity to reach a change of emphasis point. While I was going through that point, Diane's feet suddenly became warm and glowing, and she informed me that she was having a "hot flash." A few seconds later she gave a great big sigh and almost fell asleep.

5. The reflected Throat chakra was now balanced with the reflected Base chakra. This proved to be much faster than I had envisaged. Diane was still half-dazed when leaving, but fortunately her husband was driving her home.

Third Treatment Session

Diane came back for treatment after two weeks. She had initially felt elated, then tired, then elated again. The eczema had become worse (she had been warned that this may occur), her bowel movement, although erratic and sometimes explosive, had been slightly calmer that before. Altogether she was encouraged. The treatment session mirrored that of the previous session, with the addition of reinforcing the reflected Base chakra energies so as to improve her general energy and vitality.

Fourth Treatment Session

One month had elapsed since the last treatment. Diane generally felt much better in herself, she had more energy, her sleeping pattern had improved, her bowel movements were far less, and she had less pain. On reflecting, I decided to highlight the Throat and Solar Plexus chakras. The Solar Plexus chakra was treated so as to aid the digestion and help build up the liver energy. The Throat chakra was balanced with the Sacral chakra successfully, there being far less sluggishness and congested within the reflected chakras.

Diane telephoned about one month later reporting that she had never felt so well. She had also cut out wheat from her diet (on my suggestion), which had considerably improved things. In retrospect, her IBS could have been simple long-term gluten sensitivity, and the symptoms could have been eased just by change of diet. However, IBS is a notoriously complicated syndrome that is often caused by stress-related stimuli. Her long-term symptoms were probably caused by a combination of the faulty diet and stress (the two often go together). There is no doubt, though, that the treatment helped considerably to strengthen her vital force generally and her immune system in particular.

Anxiety and Depression
History

Dale, age twenty-four, was referred to me by the local general physician. He had suffered from anxiety and depression for the past ten years, ever since his mother had died in a car accident. Dale was a wiry, almost emaciated character who was frightened to the point of being phobic of needles. Acupuncture, therefore, was not on the agenda, and I decided to use the Chakra reflexology approach with a view to working on the body at a later time. The anxiety syndrome had slowly taken a hold on him over the years, and Dale often had panic attacks when in an enclosed space. He was attempting to wean himself off diazepam but was still taking antidepressants. The aim of the treatment was to "clear the wood to get to the trees" and to get to the memory cells in his system that had been so badly affected by his trauma. Dale had received no hypnotherapy or cognitive psychotherapy, which astonished me.

First Treatment Session

Shortly after the initial foot and lower-leg massage, it was clear that Dale was going to take to reflexology like a duck to water. He relaxed extremely well and was obviously confident of his surroundings and environment. Analysis during the chakra balancing stage showed there to be an imbalance in the Brow and Heart chakras (no surprise there!). The dilemma for me was which chakra to treat. I could reinforce the Brow or Heart, but on this occasion I decided to treat the Base chakra, so as to build up his vital force and to create a more generally balanced system. The Base chakra is always affected in chronic conditions and also in those syndromes related to fear of any kind.

Dale's feet were cold initially but soon came "alive" during the treatment. The Base chakra did not take too much work in order to create a balance of energy. It was during the phase of balancing the reflected Base chakra with the reflected Crown chakra that the "sigh" occurred. Following the session, Dale appeared to be much calmer. His father telephoned the following morning to report that Dale had slept like a baby and was feeling better.

Second Treatment Session

I saw Dale three days later. He had felt less anxious but paradoxically had felt more on edge and fearful, since the treatment had brought some emotional baggage to the surface. Yet Dale was willing to try anything to get well. Following the chakra balancing, I decided to treat the Heart chakra (since he had responded so well before). During the treatment, he complained of feeling very edgy and nervous—even shaky. He made a conscious effort to relax, though, and did extremely well under the circumstances. While I was finally balancing the reflected Heart chakra with the reflected Base chakra, Dale suddenly started to cry. The crying was quite violent, and I was forced to stop the treatment and sit him up over the side of the couch. It took several minutes for him to regain his composure. I advised him to rest for the remainder of the day.

Third Treatment Session

I saw Dale four days later. There had been a remarkable change in his persona. He was coherent in his speech (before he had mumbled) and was much happier in himself. He had had a few nightmares but, apart from that, he had felt much freer from the "burden inside his head." Analysis showed that the Brow chakra needed treatment, and this was duly done. I asked Dale to telephone a few days later. This he did, reporting that he knew "in his heart" that the depression and anxiety had lifted. Dale was cheerful and was actively seeking employment.

There was little doubt that reflexology with the chakra system had worked very well in this case. The added advantage of this approach over all the others is that it helps to ground the patient enough so that the true causes of the condition can be discovered.

Rheumatoid Arthritis
History

Clare, age seventy-six, had recently moved in to the area and had heard about me from another patient. She had previously been receiving regular reflexology treatments, which had "kept her going." Although she was quite happy to receive any form of therapy, I decided to stay with the reflexology approach. Her arthritis was extensive, affecting the neck, shoulders, elbows, and hands in particular. She was on constant anti-inflammatory and analgesic drugs, without which she would not be able to "function."

First Treatment Session

Following the foot massage and chakra balancing, which had highlighted the Base chakra, Solar Plexus chakra, and Throat chakra as being those in need of treatment, I decided to concentrate on treating the Base chakra. The reflected Base chakra should be the first one that is considered in all chronic illness. The patient remarked on the "different" approach, and sweetly said, "Surely it could not have any affect at all, as you aren't actually doing anything!" I would be a millionaire if every patient who had made this remark had paid me a dollar! She found the experience "relaxing" and thanked me for my trouble. Her body language suggested that she had been disappointed with my approach and would let me know if she required further treatment. This was disappointing to me but "you can't win them all." Two days later, Clare telephoned to say that she had been feeling better in herself and that the "old joints" had been just a bit easier and could she please come back for more treatment.

Second Treatment Session

I decided once again to treat the Base chakra plus, if there was enough time, the Solar Plexus. Fortunately, the next patient had cancelled, allowing sufficient time to treat both. Although it was a long session, Clare was not too uncomfortable lying on the couch but was quite stiff when the session ended. She made a further appointment for two weeks time.

Third Treatment Session

Clare reported that she had actually reduced the number of "those horrible" anti-inflammatory drugs and that her shoulders in particular seemed freer. She could undertake many more functional tasks since her last treatment and had found that filling the kettle, opening the door, and tying shoe laces were now tolerable. She was still bemused that this could have been achieved by seemingly doing nothing but touching points on the feet. This session was spent in reinforcing the reflected Base chakra and treating the Throat chakra, which had been highlighted.

Clare continued to attend at approximately monthly intervals and became a convert to my methods. With a condition such as chronic rheumatoid arthritis, we are not looking for a cure. All one can hope for is for the patient to have more functional and less painful joints. She is still progressing and even wrote of her experiences in a popular magazine. Clare still doesn't understand the treatment though!

CHAPTER FIVE

Healing

It is within the realm of "healing" that the use of the chakra energy system is best known to the general public. Later in the chapter, we will explore in detail both the hands-on and hands-off approaches to healing, based, again, on my own experiential study of more than a quarter century. First, however, let us turn to the topic of healing in general. A great deal of mystique (and ignorance) surround this simple seven-letter word.

AN OVERVIEW

An amazing thirst for knowledge on all topics allied to healing, complementary medicine, and spirituality has mushroomed over the past few years. The word *healing* simply means "to make whole." It does *not* mean "to cure." There are many aspects and types of healing. Each one, though, has a common denominator—the patient heals himself with his own complex subtle energy system. All the healer does is to provide the correct stimulus and positive thought processes to allow healing to occur.

The process of recognizing that one has a natural gift for helping one's fellow human may be long and tortuous. Many deny this inclination, putting it aside for several years, but eventually driven to it by a still, small voice that keeps whispering to them. Although it is true that everyone is capable of providing certain types of healing, I believe that a genuine gift of healing is given to one at birth and, as with any vocation, should be used. The individual concerned does not always know what kind of healing is meant for them. This part of the journey is often a matter of trial and error." Conversely, some people know exactly where their vocational gifts lie but do not know if they are to use them full-time or in their spare time while holding down another job.

The many aspects to healing may be categorized as either non-contact or contact healing. Examples of noncontact healing are: counseling, hypnotherapy, psychotherapy, radionics and radiesthesia, feng shui, distance healing, Reiki, spiritual healing, sound therapy, color therapy, magnet therapy and crystal therapy. Also in this group are therapies that heal by producing homeostasis in a person's life force, for example, homeopathy, herbal medicine, and allopathic drugs (never underestimate the power of the placebo effect).

Examples of contact healing (which does not always involve touching the physical body) may be divided into those healing professions that require a long course of study before one can achieve professional status and those that may be performed by nonprofessional therapists. Examples of the first type would include physical therapy, osteopathy, chiropractor, reflexology, craniosacral therapy, as well as shiatsu, polarity therapy, therapeutic touch, applied kinesiology, Bowen technique, acupuncture and acupressure, and massage in its myriad forms. Scores more could be included.

All the above represent types of healing, whether or not they are perceived by the therapist as such. With every type, there is an attempt to make the patient whole.

It is, however, the last category of nonprofessional contact healing that most people would consider to be "true" healing. This does not mean that some people in this category do not work as professionals, and I am not trying to discriminate or to be condescending in any way. Each person is an individual on her own life path, doing what she feels is comfortable and should not be judged by others, just because she may be doing something "different." Discrimination of the worst kind is often shown by ignorant people whose culture and belief systems clash with those of healers who are merely attempting to give love and empathy to people who need it. This final category may be subdivided into two modalities:

Magnetic healing. This is simply the ability to offer comfort to someone by placing your hands over an area of pain or congestion. Most people are capable of doing this. Self-healing mostly uses this technique. It is said that each hand, and the individual fingers, possesses either a negative, positive, or neutral magnetic influence, so placing both hands around a painful region will create a "closed circuit" of healing energy (life force, chi, prana, and so on).

Catalyst healing. This is the transference to someone, via the healer, of the natural healing power of the universe. This may be called universal life force, God, Holy Spirit, angelic beings, and so on, depending on the culture of and philosophy held by the healer. Healing may affect all levels of the person (physical, etheric, emotional, mental, or spiritual) and may be directed on-body or off-body via the chakras or through a strict protocol of positions, as in Reiki. Although healing is sometimes aimed at individual parts of the body and the symptoms that presented, this kind of healing is usually holistic in its approach. This type of healing would also include a type of Christian healing, with the minister, priest or layperson using a "laying on of hands." Many Christians believe that the healer is a channel of the power of the Holy Spirit and is using one of the "gifts of the Spirit." Obviously, healing is not just a "Christian" prerogative. Other denominations and creeds practice their own types of healing.

From the above discussion, you realize what a complicated, contentious, and emotive topic this is. This complicated study, though, is far removed from the actual practicalities of contact and noncontact healing, both of which are easy to perform. One of the dilemmas of the individual who feels that he has some kind of gift is how to nurture it so as to "answer the call." Even the most gifted and naturally inclined healer has to learn the nuts and bolts. Perhaps the first port of call would be to see a local healer or Reiki practitioner to put one's toes in the water, so to speak. The other way is to contact one of the many associations of healing.

What I attempt to do in this chapter is to offer a way for you to use contact and noncontact healing through the powerful energy centers called chakras. This system has worked well for me, and I trust that it will work well for you. First let's examine the differences between contact and noncontact chakra healing.

Frequently Asked Questions

When the therapist chooses healing as the "therapy" of choice with the chakra energy system, the dilemma is always to perform contact or noncontact healing. The FAQs at workshops are:

- Are they the same? Is one method better than the other?
- What do most therapists prefer?
- Which one would suit me?

- Can I really be doing healing if I am using contact work, which is more like acupressure?
- Will I feel awkward waving my arms around in front of a patient when she has come for "physical" therapy?

I will address all these questions over the course of this chapter. If you still have a question, though, please do not hesitate to contact me through my website. Below is a resume of the differences, advantages, and disadvantages of contact and noncontact healing. These lists, however, are by no means exhaustive.

Contact Healing

- This approach will suit the hands-on physical therapist, since there is not a huge leap of practice and philosophy between acupressure and healing.
- The therapist is comfortable, seated down most of the time with the arms relaxed
- Often, but not always, the patient accepts the idea of contact healing more readily than noncontact, since he or she feels somewhat more in control of the treatment.
- The techniques are easier to perform than those required by off-body work.
- Although this method is not as powerful and may require more time to treat a condition, this is more than compensated for by the ease of application.

Noncontact Healing

- Since most energy imbalances emanate from the subtle bodies, you are treating the true cause of the condition.

- This approach takes much more time to learn and perfect.
- There may appear to be certain anomalies in the treatment approach, and it may be difficult for the beginner to ascertain what exactly she or he is feeling.
- This approach is very subtle and takes time to learn and assimilate.
- The use of intuition is more important with this approach.
- It is often more uncomfortable for the therapist to administer, since positions need to be held for several minutes, which may lead to pain and tension in the shoulders.
- When mastered, though, this approach is ultimately more powerful and reaps greater rewards.

My advice to you if you are still feeling your way with this approach is to learn and master the contact approach before proceeding to the noncontact one. It is very important that you learn to *walk before you run.* Never attempt too much too soon—if you do, you will convey awkwardness and clumsiness to the patient. Build up confidence in one approach first. Above all, do what is comfortable for you. If you have been a physical, hands-on practitioner since training, there is no need to change. If, however, you are already been used to giving Reiki or using the subtle bodies, then noncontact therapy may be the ideal tool for you.

ANALYSIS

The first priority in healing with the chakras is to ascertain which energy centers need to be treated. As you gather information during the initial consultation, you will gain a good idea of which chakra needs attention just by the signs and symptoms presented. This meeting, though, does not give the whole picture. One of my favorite expressions is "never judge a book by its cover." This is very true when it comes to analysis and diagnosis of a patient's true imbalance. Not every patient is 100 percent truthful or open with you when reciting their symptoms and history. This is not necessarily a willful act on their part; it is just that some symptoms are much more pertinent than others. Seldom do the presenting symptoms mirror the actual cause of the condition, and it is the *cause* that you are interested in. Therefore, there has to be some other way of analyzing which system is in a state of imbalance and subsequently which chakra needs to be treated.

It has to be emphasized that assessment and "diagnosis" need to be done prior to treatment because it gives purpose to the treatment and prevents you from floundering. The patient will want to be involved in this stage and will be keen to know where the energy imbalances are. In healing, you can use two main methods, employing the *listening posts* of the cranial base or the heels and *energy balancing* the chakras prior to treatment. In both cases, only the major chakras will be discussed.

Listening Posts

Listening posts are those areas of the body that allow the practitioner to "tune in" to the various energy imbalances occurring within the body. Many parts of the body may be used, such as the shoulders (one of my favorites), knees, ankles, or various acupoints on the skull, although for practical reasons, the cranial base and heels are the ones most commonly used. The vault hold is often used as the initial hold in craniosacral therapy to ascertain the flow (or lack thereof) of the cerebrospinal fluid, whereas the heel hold is a favorite with reflexologists, merely because they are working on that part of the anatomy. Because using the heels in analysis was already discussed in Chapter 4, I will describe only the cranial base (or vault) hold here.

Vault Hold

Although you do not need to have been trained in some type of cranial therapy (craniosacral, cranial osteopathy, Indian head massage, acupressure, and so on), it would be an advantage to have practiced the basics of the procedure before using this system in analyzing the chakras. A particularly deft touch is required. Position yourself seated, behind the patient (see Figure 5.1), with him or her in a supine position with the head supported on some type of firm and supportive cushion. Place your hands under the occiput, with the little fingers

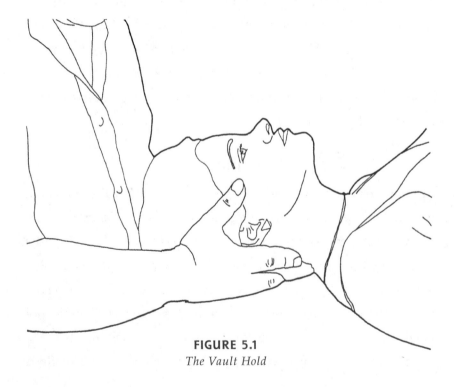

FIGURE 5.1
The Vault Hold

almost touching each other. Make sure that your forearms and elbows are supported on the couch; otherwise fatigue will set in.

The contact must be light and "airy," with no pressure whatsoever placed on the patient's skull. Nothing will happen for approximately thirty seconds to a minute, so you will need to be patient. At this point a certain amount of warmth will be created under the hands—this is merely conductive body heat. The patient may squirm a little until he or she is settled. Never be in a hurry, and never attempt to speed things on.

After approximately one to two minutes a "cranial rhythm" should be felt. This is a naturally occurring rhythm of the cerebrospinal fluid (CSF) flow. There are many schools of thought as to exactly what is being felt—some authorities insist that it is the physical movement of the CSF, whereas others would say that it is the flow of chi or vital force. I believe that in this context, *it does not really matter;* please interpret the sensations in any way that you feel comfortable with. The cranial rhythm varies between six and twenty cycles per minute, and the sensations felt under the hands are like a subtle expansion and contraction. This energetic sensation can be likened to the movement of the tide on a beach—it is in constant flow. It is important that you feel this rhythm for a few minutes before you begin with the analysis. Your brain should be "in neutral" as much as possible during this phase. By now, you should feel a warm rhythmical pulsation under your hands. After a short while, a definite shift of emphasis will be perceived. As explained in earlier chapters, this is when yours and the patient's vital forces are resonating in the alpha-theta (A/T) frequency at approximately eight cycles per second. Once this has been reached, the task of "body dowsing" and "tuning in" can be commenced—*and not before.*

The next phase of analysis using the vault hold involves the use of thought and intention. These are both powerful tools and can be quite manipulative, so it is best to use them wisely and with deference to the task in hand. Now you ask questions about the patient's chakra energy system. On no account should you speak aloud or obviously change your hand position to suggest to the patient that something is occurring. Be sure to ask yes-or-no questions; it simply does not work to ask obscure questions that would yield fuzzy answers.

Begin by asking the patient's energy system if the Base chakra is in a state of imbalance or if it needs treatment. When the answer to the question is yes, it *is* in a state of imbalance, the rhythm will appear to stop or stall. It will recommence after a few seconds, and the state of the Sacral chakra may be ascertained. Each time the rhythm ceases is an indication that an imbalance is occurring and that treatment is required. When the flow continues, this indicates that the chakra is in a state of balance and does not require treatment. You may find that two or even three chakras require treatment. There should be enough time in one hour-long treatment session to cover the analysis and up to three chakra treatments.

Chakra Balancing

Although chakra balancing is strictly another method of analysis, it may be construed as an integral part of the treatment process, and as such, is probably a more useful tool than the vault hold. One school of thought holds that energy balancing should always precede treatment in every circumstance, and in the case of healing, these are my sentiments as well. The major chakras are balanced by using the whole of the hands, or at least as much of your hand as may safely be placed on the patient's body.

Procedure

The patient needs to be sitting on the side of a couch or chair or be lying on his or her side on the couch. There has to be easy access to the anterior and posterior aspects of the body at the same time. The best way is to your patient sit on the edge of the couch; this affords ease of access. Always tell your patient what is about to happen— never "sneak" up on him or her. The "batting order" of balancing is not important, but common sense dictates that the lower major chakras should be balanced first. There are two aspects to chakra balancing—front with back and top with bottom:

Balancing front with back (anterior with posterior). Starting with the Sacral chakra, place your hands on the anterior and posterior aspect of each chakra, finishing with the Brow chakra. Under no circumstances should the anterior and posterior aspects of the Base chakra be balanced. Strictly speaking, there is only one point in any case, but two points exist for ease of access when using the chakra system with therapies. There is also only one point for the Crown chakra. You should know the exact acupoint so that you will be able to place the hands directly over the chakras, with the acupoint as the focal point. A very light touch is required and, if desired, can be done through clothes. The exception to this is that large, buckled belts need to be removed; try to ensure that just one layer of clothing is over the skin. You must be comfortable either in sitting or standing mode.

Balancing is *not* treatment—just the overture to it—therefore there is no need to keep the hand in place until a change of emphasis (A/T state) occurs. One minute is usually all that's required to create a *superficial* balance between the anterior and posterior aspects of each chakra. Energy balancing in this context means that there is a similarity of sensation under both hands. If, after about one minute, nothing appreciable is occurring under the hands, or the left hand is cold and the right one warm, or the left hand is pulsing and the right hand quiet, then a superficial energy balance *is not going to occur.* This is an indication that an imbalance exists within the chakra and *it needs treatment.* Repeat this procedure with the Solar Plexus, Heart, Throat, and Brow chakras. If the chakra balances within about a minute, it does not need to be treated. On a purely practical note, take care when balancing the Heart and Brow chakras. The anterior aspect of the Heart chakra is at CON 17 in the center of the sternum. With female patients, it is prudent to touch this point with the fingertips only—for obvious reasons. With the Brow center, although the whole hand may be placed over the two aspects, it is probably more comfortable to use the finger pads. When the front-to-back balancing has been completed, you will already have a rough indication of which chakras need to be treated, and in what order, since the most congested ones need to be tackled first.

Balancing top to bottom. Now that the anterior and posterior aspects of the chakras have been balanced one to the other, you can now balance top to bottom with the patient in supine lying if that is more comfortable, since only the anterior aspects of the chakras need be balanced. As stated before, this procedure is as much a part of the initial aspect of treatment as it is analytical. Using exactly the same pressure with the hands as before (very gentle touch), balance the anterior aspect of the chakras in the following order: Heart with Solar Plexus, Throat with Sacral, Brow with Base, and finally Crown with Base. Please be careful (for obvious reasons) when placing the hand over the Base and Heart chakras. Always make a point of both telling the patient what is about to happen, but also of getting their permission to place the hand on certain parts of their anatomy. If you are in any doubt about whether your patient will feel comfortable with having these point treated, get a chaperone to be in the room with you. After the two sets of balancing, it should be apparent which ones need to be treated, which can take place immediately with no apparent break in continuity.

CONTACT HEALING WITH THE MAJOR CHAKRAS

In Chapter 3, we explored treating the major chakras using the contact discipline of acupressure. We discussed the use of associated meridians, coupled chakras, Key points, reflex points, and other acupoints that could be used as backup and reinforcement to the treatment. When treating the major chakras in "healing" mode, the only thing that you need to know is the anatomical positioning of the chakra and its coupled chakra. Therefore, once you know the anterior and posterior positions of the major chakras, that is all that is required. The rest is up to your intuition and sensitivity of touch.

It takes time to learn this approach. It will not happen overnight. Many budding therapists who have amazing natural gifts have been put off by the seemingly lack of feel under their hands. I have encountered this regularly while running experiential workshops. It is often said that the simplest things in life take the longest to learn. It is certainly true in the world of mathematics that the easiest formulas are the hardest to prove. So it is with healing with the chakra energy system. It takes time, perseverance, and hard work to become adept and to produce results for your clients and patients. That being said, the techniques are extremely easy in practice. There is a maximum of three holds for each chakra that is in a state of imbalance, and often just two holds are required to create homeostasis:

1. Place one hand over the anterior aspect and the other hand over the posterior aspect of the chakra.
2. Place one hand over the anterior aspect of the chakra and the other hand over the coupled chakra.
3. Place one hand over the anterior aspect of the chakra and the other on the Crown chakra.

Treating the Anterior and Posterior Aspects of the Affected Chakra

In Chapter 2, I stated that a person's chakras, their gateway to communion with the spiritual and other subtle auric bodies, lie all around the body at a certain level of the spine and torso. The anterior and posterior aspects on the midline of the body are merely the focal areas that have, historically, been used by clairvoyants, healers, yogi, gurus, Sufi masters, and others involved in the healing arts. It is, therefore, these two areas that are used in practice, although *any* part of the circle of energy could be used if needed. I make this important point at this juncture to explain that if contact or noncontact healing through the recognized chakras does not yield the desired results, then you may find another area on the same level that will fit the bill. In everyday practice this is a rare occurrence, but I have known it to happen.

The patient should be either in side or supine lying. It is all a question of personal comfort for both parties. If your patient is lying on his side, your arms may start to get tired, so you may prefer to stand. With the patient lying supine, your hand under the patient may (for a few minutes) take quite a lot of their body weight. This is particularly true with the posterior Heart, Solar Plexus, and Base chakras. The posterior Throat and Sacral chakra holds do not take as much weight. The posterior Sacral chakra is situated at the upper aspect of the lumbar lordosis, and it is easy to slide the hand underneath. Of the two positions, supine lying treatment is easier to perform. Patients are much more comfortable in that position, and it is generally easier on the practitioner. Because of the nature of the holds, your forearm has to rest on the client.

When treating the Base chakra, the underneath hand is gently manipulated under the patient's bottom, with the fingertips on the underside of the coccyx. The top hand rests over the symphysis pubis. Although this can be a "delicate" procedure, once the treatment has started, all thoughts of the actual anatomical positioning are forgotten. Please note that the "under-sacrum" hold that is used in craniosacral therapy is not adopted in this instance. Fingertips are usually used with the Brow chakra, since this saves placing the whole hand over the patient's eyes (unlike in Reiki). Since there is only one point for the Crown chakra, treatment in contact healing mode needs to be approached differently. The easiest way is for you to be seat at your client's head, with him or her in a comfortable position and to place both hands on the top of the skull, with the tips of the middle fingers being opposed and Gov 20 in between. The skin is gently stretched, but essentially the fingers keep still.

As with other methods of contact work, nothing will be felt initially, and it will take well over a minute for the patient to relax onto the hands. You will then feel warmth for another couple of minutes. By now, though, you should start to feel the imbalance, that is, a "sluggishness" will be felt in the congested chakra, and a "fizzing" should be felt in a hyperactive chakra. Please note that the congested state is by far the most common to be treated. After about four minutes or so have elapsed, you should feel a change of emphasis under your hands. When in acupressure mode, this is the signal for the treatment to end and for you to continue with other acupoints. In healing mode, however, it is the signal that the treatment has just *commenced*. The hands should be quite still, although if the patient appears to be moving slightly, then follow these movements with your hands.

Your thoughts and intentions are very important, especially at this critical stage of the procedure. Try not to have any extraneous thoughts, and keep focused on the job at hand. Above all, do not try to "will" anything to happen—keep an open mind. You will be receiving constant feedback through your hands, and this has to be interpreted. Within the next few minutes, the sensations under the hands may change. What was once very sluggish (in a subtle sense) will slowly become less heavy, more permeable, and lighter in nature and texture. The breakthrough can occur very slowly or almost instantaneously—each case is different. What normally occurs at this time is that the patient will take a huge breath, sigh, or yawn and will feel very much more relaxed afterward. Occasionally, an emotional outburst can occur (have tissues on hand). The two of you have now reached the point where the chakra is starting to clear of congestion. The hold should be continued, though, for a couple more minutes until nothing else is occurring under the hands. To sum up, the sensations that could be felt under the hands are, in order:

1. nothing at all
2. warmth by conductive heat
3. a heavy "porridge like" sensation
4. a lighter and airier state—through the A/T state

5. warmth, clarity, and lightness

6. a blissful state and a feeling of endlessness

It is now time to remove the underneath hand (sometimes a blessed relief) to do the next part of the treatment.

Balancing the Affected Chakra with Its Coupled Chakra

Once the chakra has been cleared by contact healing, it is now time to balance it with its coupled chakra. The reason for this is that the chakra often becomes imbalanced because of the coupled chakra's influence, and this imbalance has to be addressed. The technique is exactly the same as it was above, with the exception that it will be quicker and you will feel more comfortable! Now that your hands are getting more adept at sensing changes in the qualities of subtle energy, you should be able to feel the differences between the energy qualities of the two centers after a few seconds. The upper body chakras will naturally feel lighter and airier by their very nature, but the task at hand is to end up with an equal sensation under both hands. Sometimes the coupled chakra is as congested as the original one. This stage of the procedure should last no more than three to four minutes. Although this section has concentrated on the anterior aspect of the chakra, if the posterior aspect is the one that needs healing, as in a chronic spinal condition, then it is *this* aspect that is worked on.

Balancing the Affected Chakra with the Crown Chakra

This last stage is not needed if (a) the Base chakra has been treated (b) the Crown chakra is being treated. In every other case, it is a good thing to energy balance the affected chakra with the Crown. This will help enormously if there is any emotional aspect to the condition (which there usually is). The Crown chakra should be held with an extremely light (almost ethereal) touch. Do not be surprised if this hold takes a little longer than the previous one. There is quite a lot of assimilation to be carried out by the patient's energy system, and it may take a couple of minutes before anything starts to happen. The whole procedure, including all three stages, should take no longer than about twenty to twenty-five minutes.

Before the patient sits up on the side of the couch, it is essential that you ask him how he is feeling. If he feels lightheaded or disoriented he must not be allowed to leave and definitely not to drive a car until he has been "grounded." This can be easily achieved by placing the middle finger pads on bilateral point KID 1 (Foot chakra) on the soles of the feet for about two minutes.

Examples of Conditions Treated in Healing Mode

Below I list some of the conditions that appear to answer to healing with the chakras and the personality traits of the people with these conditions. The personality traits are not conditions per se; rather, they represent a symptomatic picture of the whole person and might be brought about by upbringing, culture, or belief system. It is often the "nearest and dearest" of the client (who frequently are present at the consultation) who will give information regarding the personality. The questions about fears and phobias aspect are very important. Try to ask questions about fear in a subtle way. Some of these are chronic physical conditions, and some are emotional. Most of the physical conditions, though, have been brought about by emotional etiology. By providing the list I do not mean to infer that any of these conditions or situations cannot be treated using other disciplines or that only emotional conditions can be treated in healing mode.

Crown Chakra Imbalance

Physical—headache, vertigo

Emotional—depression, delusion, illusion, erratic mood swings, melancholy, phobias

Personality and Characteristics—strong, courageous, truthful, proud, ambitious, arrogant, controlling, obstinate, intolerant, angry, impatient, unsympathetic, immoral—*fear of exposure and guilt* (a common reason for suicide)

Brow Chakra Imbalance

Physical—migraine, vertigo, catarrh

Emotional—anger, rage, indecision, and indifference

Personality and Characteristics—self-centered, lacking in moral courage, passionate, changeable, seeking and searching, discontent, conflicted within, obsessed—*fear of stagnation and stillness*

Throat Chakra Imbalance

Physical—chronic sore throat, constipation, frozen shoulder, cervical spondylosis

Emotional—shyness, introversion, paranoia, anxiety

Personality and Characteristics—insecure, critical, selfish, materialistic, suppressed emotionally, agoraphobic, unwilling to change direction, proud, isolated, absentminded, perfectionistic, repressed—*phobic fears*

Heart Chakra Imbalance

Physical—chronic heart and circulation conditions

Emotional—tearful, anxious, detached, depressed

Personality and Characteristics—indifferent to and contemptuous of others' mental limitations, suffering from inferiority complex, self-pitying, claustrophobic, unable to show and give love, constantly anxious about self—*fear of showing emotions*

Solar Plexus Chakra Imbalance

Physical—allergies, chronic fatigue, stomach and liver conditions

Emotional—depression, anxiety, self-pity, panic, worry

Personality and Characteristics—narrow-minded, obsessed with past events, reluctant to change, rigid in thoughts and belief systems, possessive, willing to serve others without reward, anxious and worried for others—*fear of insecurity*

Sacral Chakra Imbalance

Physical—sexual conditions, edema

Emotional—jealousy, envy, lust

Personality and Characteristics—reverent, devotional, proud, lacking in self-esteem, poor at communication and relationships, prone to deep depressions, critical, indulgent in fantasy—*fear of failure*

Base Chakra Imbalance

Physical—kidney and chronic spinal conditions

Emotional—insecurity, doubt, mind in turmoil

Personality and Characteristics—rigid, ritualistic, superstitious, proud, opinionated, obsessive, unable to ground self, changeable, lonely, fearful of change, attracted to glamour, bigoted, ecstatic, insanity— *fear of madness*

CONTACT HEALING WITH THE MINOR CHAKRAS

Although it is generally accepted that only the major chakras possess a link to the etheric, emotional, mental, and spiritual realms of the individual, there is no doubt in my mind that the minor chakras can also affect at least the first three subtle bodies. When you use the same approach as you did with the majors, the results obtained can be of enormous significance. Minor chakras may be treated in healing mode as individual areas or in combination with the coupled major chakra. Below are examples of how the minor chakra system may be used in healing mode, along with some relevant conditions. These are placed in anatomical order from the top downward:

1. Ear chakras
2. Shoulder chakras
3. Elbow chakras
4. Hand chakras
5. Knee chakras
6. Foot chakras

There is no reason why the others, such as the Clavicular, Intercostal, Navel, and Groin chakras, may not be treated in healing mode, although since they are associated so strongly with the relevant major chakras, further consideration here is not warranted.

Ear Chakras

Examples of Conditions—hardness of hearing, tinnitus, TMJ syndrome, grief

With the patient lying supine, position yourself behind his or her head. Gradually introduce the pads of the middle fingers to both TE 17 points, just behind the lobes of the ear. As with all holds that need to be maintained over a period of time, make sure your forearms are well supported. The sensations felt should be exactly the same as those experienced while treating a major chakra; the hold could take about twenty minutes total. The patient may experience all kinds of "weird and wonderful" sensations in the ears and head during this time, and you will feel, after a short while, that your fingers are not in contact at all; it will all begin to feel quite ethereal. When you are sure that the treatment is concluded, try to energy balance with the Ear chakra's major chakra couple—the Heart chakra. This should be carried out especially with emotional conditions such as grief. Just one of the two Ear chakra points need be used in the balance.

Shoulder Chakras

Examples of Conditions—shoulder and neck tension, constipation, shyness and introversion, suppressed emotions, and an inability to be "free"

As with the Ear chakras, the bilateral Shoulder chakra points are approached from behind the head of the supine-lying patient. They are best treated with the whole hand over the shoulders with the focal point (middle of the palm) over the LI 15 acupoint. Shoulder chakra treatment is a wonderful way of reducing tension (especially in the neck and trapezius muscles) and of easing general body tension. Much tension can build up around the shoulder region over a period of many years. This often leads to cervical and upper thoracic conditions, as well as fibrositis and capsulitis of the joint. People who worry a lot about themselves and others have a tendency to have shoulder tension, as do people who cannot express themselves (physically and emotionally). A very light touch should be employed, with the hands hardly in contact. Once the various levels of the healing treatment have been concluded to your satisfaction, try to lift the hands off the body about half an inch to start the experiment into etheric and off-body healing. Leave the hands in place for a few minutes and gauge the difference—more about this later in the chapter. Once the treatment has concluded, you may energy balance the Shoulder chakra with either the coupled major—the Throat chakra or the coupled minor—or the Navel chakra, depending on the symptoms presented.

Elbow Chakras

Examples of Conditions—Chronic tennis and /golfer's elbow or joint capsulitis, cervical tension, lack of assertiveness, inflexibility, and resentfulness toward others.

You now have to sit at the patient's side to properly place the hands on the Elbow chakras. It may mean that your forearm will be resting on his abdominal region, unless he can rest his own arms on his front. The finger pads or the whole hand may be used in this hold. Elbows are areas where, once again, much tension may be stored. People who are resentful, jealous, envious of others often develop elbow conditions. Shy and diffident people who have difficulty in showing their feelings are also troubled in this region. The treatment may be concluded by balancing with the coupled minor chakra—the Knee chakra or the coupled major chakra, the Base chakra.

Hand Chakras

Examples of Conditions—General stiffness and/or arthritic changes; resistance to expressing feelings, too much criticism of self and others; being withdrawn and reclusive.

The bilateral Hand chakras may be treated with the whole of the hand placed underneath the patient's hands or with the pads of the middle fingers placed on top. Do what is comfortable. Hand chakra healing is very effective and usually quite quick to do. The patient may inform you that, as the healing progresses, her head feels clearer. This is quite normal, since the Hand chakra causes the head to clear when it is used in acupressure mode, as opposed to when it is used in healing mode. Treatment may be rounded off by balancing with the coupled minor chakra—the Foot chakra or the coupled major chakra, the Crown chakra.

Knee Chakras

Examples of Conditions—Chronic knee stiffness and/or arthritic changes, stubbornness, pride, arrogance

In her book *Your Body Speaks Your Mind*, Debby Shapiro writes of the knees:

> The knees are like shock absorbers, taking the strain between the weight of the body above and the ups and downs of the terrain below. When we can't bear the load any more, the knees may start to react. They are telling us to relax, to find our flow again, to let go of the pressure. Water on the knee indicates a holding of emotional energy,

particularly a resistance to surrender; or there may be too much emotion to cope with and the weight is being carried in the knees. An inflamed knee indicates that something or someone is making us irritated or angry, and we will not give in!

Healing may be given (as with all the other joints) to just one joint or to both at the same time. Individual joints are healed by placing one hand on either side of the joint and going through the various layers and levels previously described. Do not forget that the influence of the chakra is all around a particular level, and the minor chakras are no exception to this. The best way to treat the knee in healing mode is to place the hands anterior and posterior of the joint. In this way, the focal point of BL 40, in the center of the popliteal fossa, may be influenced. When treating both knees, place the hands underneath the patient's knees, with him or her lying supine or sitting. On completion of the healing, you may balance the Knee chakra with the coupled minor—the Elbow chakra or the coupled major, the Base chakra.

Foot Chakra

Examples of Conditions—Chronic ankle and foot stiffness and arthritis, bunions, unsureness of life's direction, anxiety and fear, the need to be grounded.

When the foot is suffering from a chronic physical condition it needs to be treated by placing one hand over the dorsum and the other hand over the plantar aspect, with the focus through KID 1, on the sole of the foot. If the person has emotional problems such as fear, anxiety, rigid belief systems, and so on, then both feet need to be treated at the same time. This may be done by placing the middle finger pads on KID 1 or by placing the palms on the patient's soles. The latter is a favorite with reflexologists when "finishing off" a treatment session. It is also a favored region to use in healing when the patient needs to be grounded, for whatever reason. When the treatment is completed, it may be balanced with the Crown or the Hand chakras.

NONCONTACT HEALING

Since this book opened with a description of the aura, it seems fitting that it be concluded with a discussion of the ways in which the aura can be manipulated and analyzed in order to use the chakras in off-body mode. Many books have been published on the subject of noncontact healing, and there are as many ideas on the topic as there are books and articles. Once again, this chapter is based purely on my own observations over three decades of using this healing system of. It is not meant to debunk or criticize any other form of noncontact healing. One point that must be stressed, however, over and over again is that budding hands-on therapists who are taking that extra leap of faith in using the aura must adopt a "softly, softly" approach. Do not expect to be able to feel everything the very first time you try it. It never ceases to amaze me that sensible practitioners realize that it takes months, if not years, to master their contact form of therapy but naturally assume that noncontact healing can be mastered in a few days! These techniques come naturally over a period of weeks, if not months. They require patience, perseverance, and a deft touch. Don't be frustrated or hasty.

The other thing to mention at this stage is that off-body healing is not everyone's cup of tea, and not everyone is meant to practice it. Do not even attempt to learn it if you are not comfortable with the idea. Some people have the misguided idea that off-body work is like waving the arms around some distance from the patient as if something mystical or divine were suddenly going to intervene. It is *nothing* like that! It is an exact and carefully monitored procedure that has a beginning, middle, and end with carefully drawn-up protocols. Please accept also that you as the practitioner are the interpreter and facilitator of the patient's own energy system. There is nothing emanating from you that influences the patient. You are not the healer; ultimately it is the person who heals him- or herself.

The Aura

Here is a brief recap of what comprises the aura and what you should feel in analysis and treatment. You may also want to reread the section about auras at the beginning of Chapter 1. The aura (or subtle bodies) is comprised of the etheric (two different layers), emotional (astral), mental, intuitional, monadic, and divine levels. They are often given different names depending on the creeds, philosophies, and cultures of those who devised them. Only the first three will be discussed in detail, since the others fall well outside the scope of this book. Table 5.1 shows the subtle body, its color according to clairvoyants, the distance away from the physical body, and what a congested chakra at this level may feel like.

In Chapter 1, I suggested that the aura could be felt by bringing the hands closely together from a distance of about two feet or so. A kind of subtle barrier should be felt when the hands are about four inches (ten centimeters) apart and a less obvious one with the hands about ten inches (twenty-five centimeters) apart. These positions are where the boundaries of the etheric and emotional bodies of the

TABLE 5.1. COLOR, DISTANCE FROM PHYSICAL BODY, AND CONGESTION SENSATIONS OF THE AURA

Auric Level	Color	Distance from Body	Sensation of Physical Congestion
Physical-Etheric	Bluish gray	Three quarters to one inch (two to three centimeters)	Dense and heavy sensation (like treacle)
Etheric-Emotional	Bluish gray—less dense	Three to four inches (eight to ten centimeters)	Slightly less dense (like water)
Emotional	Bluish yellow	Ten to twelve inches (twenty-five to thirty centimeters)	"Fizzing" or "buzzing"
Mental	Whitish yellow	Up to two and a half feet (seventy-five centimeters)	Mini electric shock Sensation of "tingling"

hands are being felt. The more you do this simple exercise, the more you will become used to the subtlety and deft touch that is required. Another exercise that you can do is called massaging, or stimulation of the aura.

Stimulation of the Aura

Aura stimulation may be carried out on a friend or on yourself—you can even teach it at workshops! Choose a stiff joint or sluggish area of the body that is easily accessible. It could be a stiff thumb, elbow, or knee, for example. Do *not* touch the body part at the beginning. The idea is to stimulate the aura above the stiff or sluggish part of the body sufficiently to make an impression on the part by improving the range of movement and decreasing the stiffness. One or both hands may be used (or more exactly, the fingertip). Simply make swirling and continuous movements between one to three inches (two to five centimeters) above the joint. Initially, neither you nor the patient will feel anything. After about half a minute, you will feel heat and a kind of heavy sensation build under the fingers, and the patient will begin to experience warmth building up in the area. Proceed in this way for about three minutes or so and see what different sensations are felt and received. When this is finished (and the part still not touched), ask the patient to move the joint. You will find that there is more movement and less pain. All that has been accomplished is that the etheric body has been sufficiently stimulated to improve the energy makeup and the blood circulation to the physical body. If this can be achieved at any area of the body, imagine what can be achieved when working through the main energy centers!

Analysis of the Auric Chakras

There are two distinct ways to gauge the state of the chakras in the subtle bodies before balance/treatment is commenced. The first way is by using the technique previously described, using the Listening Posts of the cranial base (occiput) or the heels. You simply "ask" the client if the aura needs balancing in whatever state you ascertained the physical aspect of the chakra to be in. It is a personal choice, of course, but the second way, described below, would be strongly recommend—that of reading the aura by feel.

Feeling the Aura

Make sure that the patient is relaxed and lying supine. Stand beside her and introduce one hand (the other is redundant for the moment) into her etheric body no more than four inches (ten centimeters) (the upper border of the etheric body) above her physical body. This *must* be carried out with great care and deference to the person on the couch. Never introduce or remove the hand quickly; otherwise, "auric shock" may occur. The hand remains quite still over the body for a few seconds until the patient is used to its presence; this will be for about ten seconds. Following this, move the hand very slowly at a constant height from the patient, stopping over the center of each chakra for a few seconds. Any chakra (major or minor, or even acupoints) can be assessed in this way, so there is no rigid start and end to the procedure. The best way, however, would be to commence at the soles of the feet with the Foot chakras, go to the Knee chakras (which may be accessed on the anterior aspect), then the Hand chakras, Elbow chakras, Shoulder chakras, then back down to the Base chakra, Groin chakras, Sacral chakra, Navel chakras, Solar Plexus chakra, Intercostal chakras, Heart chakra, Throat chakra, Clavicular chakras, Ear chakras, Brow chakra, and finally Crown chakra. It does not matter in which order this procedure is carried out, as long as each chakra is carefully monitored. When you are new to this way of working, you should stick to monitoring the major chakras only until you feel confident about doing them all.

When an imbalance exists in a chakra at the etheric level, it feels more "sluggish" than the surrounding aura. In the table above, I used the expressions "dense and heavy" and "less dense and heavy" to describe a congested physical-etheric and etheric-emotional chakra, respectively. It is very difficult to adequately describe in words alone the sensations that are felt. There are so many comparisons that could be made. I have heard them described as "pea soup," "oil," or even "earth." The most important thing to remember is that it is the comparison of each chakra that matters. It is often a good idea to go through the procedure twice so as to make absolutely sure that what is felt is real. You can be fooled very easily if your total focus is not on the task in hand.

Chakra Size and Other Subtle Bodies

Taking into account that each person is different, you should know the average size of the chakras so that you can be accurate in the analysis and treatment modes. The chakra has been described as an inverted ice cream cone with the single acupoint on the physical body flowering out into a whirling vortex of energy. At the physical-etheric upper level of approximately three quarters of an inch, the chakra is roughly the diameter of two and a half inches. Since this circle is relatively small, the finger pads of the middle fingers are normally used in assessment and/or treatment. At the etheric-emotional upper level of about four inches, the diameter is about three and a half to four inches, the average diameter of a mug. At the outer level of the emotional body, ten inches from the physical, the chakra diameter is roughly the size of a small plate, the diameter of six inches. You should have easily deduced by now that quite a bit of overlapping of the major chakras occurs beyond the etheric level. At the upper extremity of the mental body, about two and a half feet above the physical body, the diameter is the size of a twelve-inch dinner plate. Knowledge of overlapping is very important, because, as discussed later, it is the individual part of the chakra that is important. You have to make sure that you are feeling the upper aspect of one chakra and not the lower aspect of the adjacent one. (See Figure 5.2.)

As table 5.1 shows, the sensation of a congested chakra feels different at its upper levels of the emotional (astral) and mental body.

When your hands are placed over four inches away from the physical body to affect the emotional body, the imbalance felt is more like a constantly moving "fizzing" sensation on the fingers. The mental body is even more pronounced, with sensations of small electric shocks or "tingles." The individual sensations do not matter, since each is a personal interpretation. What *is* important is the comparison of the sensation of each chakra at the same vertical height above the physical body. You do not need to assess the chakras at every level if the etheric is found to be imbalanced, but it is a good habit to

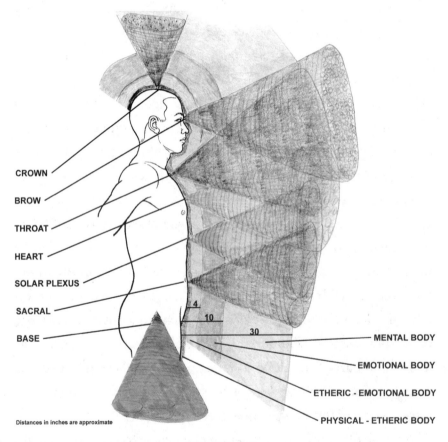

CROWN
BROW
THROAT
HEART
SOLAR PLEXUS
SACRAL
BASE

4
10
30

MENTAL BODY
EMOTIONAL BODY
ETHERIC - EMOTIONAL BODY
PHYSICAL - ETHERIC BODY

Distances in inches are approximate

FIGURE 5.2

Diagrammatic Interpretation of Overlapping Chakras above Emotional Body

adopt, because the treatment that follows will rely on good analysis and assessment of the whole of the chakra.

Nature of the Chakra

If everything that has been described in the previous section is not enough to boggle your mind, the natural vibration of each chakra needs also to be taken into account when analyzing the whole chakra. As mentioned earlier, in each chakra there are four or more components of rotating vortices that form smaller chakras, and they themselves seem to be roughly cylindrical in shape. It is these individual components where clairvoyants have perceived vibrations at certain frequencies. The lower chakras resonate somewhat slowly, while the Brow and Crown chakras resonate at a phenomenal rate. These differences should be taken into account as part of the whole analytical package. It is said that the Base chakra consists of four rotating vortices, the Sacral chakra has six, the Solar Plexus chakra has ten, the Heart chakra has twelve, the Throat chakra has sixteen, the Brow chakra has ninety-six, and the Crown chakra has a staggering 972. (See Color Plates 2–8 showing the clairvoyants view of the chakras).

As well as being divided into four or more whirling spherical components, it is said that each chakra has a central "core" with radiating segments, rather like the cornea and iris in the eye. It all appears to be very complicated, and some people are put off by the whole idea of off-body work because of this. It was, indeed, a real struggle when I was first introduced to the intricacies and convolutions of the chakra system. All is not lost, however. What I have earnestly sought over many years of teaching this approach is to make the whole concept of chakra healing (with all modalities) accessible to the average practitioner. This has necessitated devising a different system of analysis and treatment of the subtle bodies that, although not easy to learn, does away with the need to learn all the other aspects.

This is not to say that everything else should be ignored, but in clinical terms the important thing to appreciate is that the lower chakras vibrate at a lower frequency and therefore naturally feel more sluggish. A congested Base chakra will feel somewhat different from a congested Brow chakra. The difference, though, is very subtle, so appreciate and accept it, but don't let it become an issue. As stated before, it is important in analysis and treatment to ascertain which part of the chakra is in a state of imbalance. Below represents my own interpretation of imbalanced major chakras based on several years of study.

Interpretation of Imbalance in the Major Chakras

The previous section outlined the different qualities that can be felt at different levels of ascertaining which of the chakras needed to be balanced and treated in healing mode. The following describes a way of looking at the auric chakra at the etheric-emotional level at about five to six inches from the physical body. I have chosen this level purposely, since beyond it overlapping occurs, and the interpretation is not as clear-cut or as easy. Figure 5.3 shows a plan of the chakra from the perspective of looking down from above. It shows an outer circle, although in reality, a somewhat imperfect circle is the true picture. The chakra is divided roughly into the positions on the hands of the clock and also into concentric circles within. From this, therefore, it is possible to accurately ascertain where, for example, outer twelve o'clock, inner nine o'clock, or middle four o'clock appear. The top of the chakra at twelve o'clock is nearest to the person's head, and the six o'clock is facing the feet. The diagram shows which aspects of the physical body are associated with each chakra and subsequently which organs are affected in chakra imbalance.

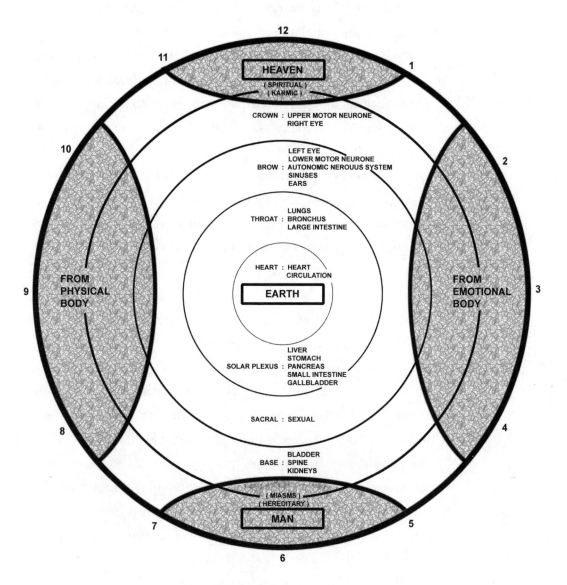

FIGURE 5.3

Interpretation of the Chakras at the Etheric/Emotional Level

The whole of the chakra is divided into the three aesthetic qualities of *heaven, earth,* and *man.* These areas show if the imbalance is
of a spiritual or "karmic" nature, represented in the heaven segment;
if the imbalance is hereditary or miasmatic, represented in the man
segment; or if the imbalance is emanating from the physical body
or from the subtler body of the emotional layer, represented by the
remainder of the chakra. The heaven segment is found around the
twelve o'clock region, the hereditary segment is found around the
six o'clock segment, if the cause of the imbalance is in the physical
body, this is felt around the nine o'clock segment, and if the cause
emanates from either the emotional or mental body, this is felt around
the three o'clock segment. This interpretation is extremely significant from a clinical viewpoint. This is how it works in practice:

1. Complete the analysis as previously detailed at the etheric and
   etheric-emotional levels. It will be found, in general terms, that
   one chakra is more "sluggish" than the others. These are the ones
   that need to be balanced and cleared (healed). It is often the case
   that the coupled chakras are also in a state of imbalance, which
   makes subsequent treatment easier.

2. The imbalanced chakras now need to be further investigated at
   the etheric-emotional level to ascertain further analysis. Should
   the twelve o'clock region be highlighted (that is, should it be more
   sluggish than any other area), this is interpreted as a condition
   that is part of the spiritual makeup (some philosophies would
   call it "karma"); very little can be done to address the true cause.
   The physical symptoms may be addressed, but not the cause.
   Some authorities believe that karma can be influenced, but this
   is well beyond both the scope of this book and beyond the capac-
   ity of my tiny brain to comprehend.

3. Should the six o'clock region be highlighted regarding the "amount" of sluggishness felt, this indicates that the condition is part of an ancestral quality that has been passed down from a previous generation. The modern terminology would be *genetic coding*, but philosophers such as Samuel Hahnemann, the founder of modern homeopathy, coined the word *miasm* to indicate the taints of disease that are inherent in our makeup.

4. Should the three o'clock region be highlighted regarding the amount of sluggishness or "action" felt under the fingers, this indicates that the cause is neither karmic nor hereditary, but that it is of one's own making, being influenced by one of the subtler bodies. It could be that one's thoughts or emotions have influenced the physical body via the chakras.

5. Should the nine o'clock region be highlighted, this indicates that, again, the condition is of one's own making. This time, the cause is emanating from the physical body. This could be personal abuse over a long period of time due to smoking, eating too many wrong foods, sexual excesses, allergic responses, or a hundred and one different causes.

6. Now, very slowly and gently, take the hand once more to the superior aspect (top) of the chakra just below the twelve o'clock segment and slowly "feel" around the chakra's main body. This indicates which part of the main bulk of the chakra is imbalanced. It must be carried out with the fingertips, sine the analysis has to be very precise. It will be found that an area (or areas) within the main body of the chakra will feel more sluggish than that of the surrounding chakra. It could be, for example, eleven o'clock outer aspect, five o'clock middle aspect, or right in the very center of the chakra. Clairvoyants and some gifted "spiritual" healers have

stated that the various anatomical positioning of the areas of sluggishness means something. Except for the four segments already mentioned, the only significance of the positioning of the individual areas of sluggishness within the chakra is that it needs to be known when it comes to treatment. Further analysis may be warranted if you feel that it will fill a void in your knowledge gap, but my feeling is that it is not worth becoming too dogmatic over the interpretation—just accept it and carry on!

TREATING THE AURIC CHAKRAS

In this section we explore the esoteric side of healing, which I imagine is what the general public considers the only way that the energy centers are used. However, we know different.

Keeping the Patient Informed

Your patient will naturally be curious about your findings and will be eager to have your interpretations revealed. Never underestimate his or her curiosity or ability to understand. If it is found that the cause of the condition is coming from the physical body, a brief explanation of possible changes in personal habits, diet, and such will help. The patient will most likely have come to the same conclusion. If the cause is emanating from the mental or emotional bodies, the explanation can be a little trickier. It could be that he or she will have to start changing their lifestyle or alter some deep-seated belief system, or it may be as simple as merely indicating that worry or stress has been the cause of the physical condition. People are generally willing to change if they are going to feel better in the long run. Patients will also readily accept the explanation of a condition being hereditary or due to genetic coding. Even though there is little chance of treating the cause (except through radical surgery, bone marrow transplant, or blood transfusion), there is every chance of easing the symptoms by methods that will be shown later.

Since we are touching on blood transfusions, it is my belief that it is possible to acquire some of the donor's miasmatic or genetic coding, which may completely change their disease process. Always ask a prospective patient as part of your questionnaire if he or she has had transplant surgery or transfusions. The one aspect that could be a little trickier in its explanation is telling the patient that the condition is part of his or her karma. Some patients are well aware of this phenomenon and accept it readily, while others definitely do not! Please tread carefully and respect their belief systems. They are also curious about what you are able to feel of their body's imbalance. Describe the sensations you feel as coherently and simply as you can, although it is not always easy to put these sensations into words.

The Physical-Etheric Body

The etheric body is found up to four inches away from the physical body. As stated before, there are two parts to it—the physical-etheric and the etheric-emotional. There is quite a difference between these two in the way they affect treatment. When congestion and sluggishness are found in the physical-etheric body, you should offer gentle stimulation of the aura at that level. This is performed by massaging the aura, as previously described. This is usually done with the fingertips of the middle fingers and with rapid circular movements. After a little while, the sluggishness appears to disappear and the whole area becomes lighter, then quite warm, then very warm, and, finally, the sensation appears to be the same as if part of the etheric had been massaged over a non congested area. The whole procedure takes a couple of minutes. This technique is ideal when the imbalance is coming from the physical body that was initiated weeks or months previously. If this be the case, the imbalance has not yet had a stranglehold on the patient, and the upper aura has not yet been affected.

The Etheric-Emotional Body

Treatment at the etheric-emotional level between two and four inches above the physical body requires a different approach. The feeling of congestion is not as dense as described in the previous section, and this needs to be appreciated. Once you locate the congested area with, say, the right hand (it could vary in size, so either locate it with the fingertip or the hand), find the *exact* same part of the coupled chakra with the other hand (or middle finger). For instance, if the three o'clock inner part of the Throat chakra is congested, then go to three o'clock inner part of the Sacral chakra. Sometimes, this area has to be gently felt for. Try not to "fish" around too much, since this will disturb the subtle energy field. The exact part of the coupled chakra should show congestion in any case, so it should be relatively easy to locate. Once you have found the two areas, keep the hands initially quite still on them for about a minute to see if the sensation changes. If it does (it should feel lighter, but don't panic if it feels more sluggish), keep your hands perfectly still until the area has cleared altogether and it has the same sensation as the parts adjacent to the hands. If the sluggishness does not clear or becomes denser, the areas need to be massaged very gently until the area starts to change. This may take up to about five minutes, which is a long time to keep the hands hovering over the body. The length of time the area takes to clear indicates the chronicity of the imbalance. You can proceed to check the chakra at the next subtle level, balance the chakra with the etheric Crown, or give a hands-on treatment. If the latter is carried out, the balance should occur quite quickly.

The Emotional Body

As stated before, the sensation of congestion within the emotional body is that of "fizzing," "water trickling," "buzzing" or one of a myriad of other sensations—that is why it is so difficult to teach this topic. The emotional body ranges from approximately four inches to about twelve inches above the physical body. Therefore, the area of imbalance to be felt for is quite substantial. The best way to ascertain where the exact point of congestion lies is to do slow, rhythmical sweeps with the dominant hand to try and "pick it up." This may take a number of seconds to achieve. Never sweep the aura with any degree of vigor or stimulation—this will only upset the auric balance. When you have found the "fizzing" or "buzzing, keep the dominant hand perfectly still, while with the other hand you find the exact area of the coupled chakra. If, for instance, the congestion is found in the outer five o'clock region of the Brow chakra, then the other hand must go to the outer five o'clock area of the Base chakra. The sensation found at the coupled chakra may not be one of "buzzing" or "fizzing." It will not, however, feel totally clear. Some form of congestion will be felt, sometimes a sensation of "cold," sometimes of "spikiness." Keep both hands in place for as long as it takes to create a sameness of sensation under both hands that also feels harmonious and comfortable. The "fizzing" sensation may disappear within seconds or may take a few minutes.

Do *not* stimulate this area; the "healing" has to be done keeping the hands perfectly still. Just before the areas clear and harmony is achieved, the patient will often respond with a sigh or yawn (assuming he or she is even awake at this juncture). The next stage is either to proceed to the mental body to ascertain whether or not imbalance exists in that body or to energy balances the previously congested area in the chakra with the emotional level of the Crown chakra. This does not have to comply with the exact positioning of the coupled chakra—the center of the Crown chakra will suffice.

The Mental Body

The mental body can be approximately twelve inches to three feet above the physical body. As stated before, the sensation of congestion is one of a slight electric shock or tingling under the fingers. As with the emotional body, ascertain the exact area of imbalance by doing gentle sweeping with the dominant hand. As you may by now be working approximately two feet above the physical body, the sensations are much subtler than those of the previous parts of the aura. Even though it feels subtler, you must always be aware that the healing achieved at this level may have profound effects on your patient. Never get lulled into a sense that you aren't achieving anything—nothing could be further from the truth. At the mental level, there is no need to balance the congested area with the coupled chakra. For once, the nondominant hand is redundant. The tingling sensation will often take a few minutes to disappear and as with the treatment of other subtle bodies is often heralded by yawning or sighing. The patient may also feel many different "weird and wonderful" sensations within her physical body. It is good thing for her to quietly discuss these with you. There should not be too much talking, since you need to focus and concentrate, but nonetheless, communication is very important. When the area has been cleared, the next stage of healing at this level is to place the dominant hand within the mental level of the Crown chakra. Tingling and "shocks" will always be felt within the Crown at this level, and you should home in on these areas. It is important to clear the Crown chakra congestion as much as possible, since this chakra, above all others, is the one true gateway to the person's higher centers and ultimately their spirituality. There is always imbalance to be found in the Crown chakra; sometimes it feels like a minefield of activity. The sensations felt, though, may not be mirrored in the physical body as symptoms.

Auric Chakras

The possibility of there being auric chakras was mentioned earlier in the book. Some authorities have indicated that there may be up to ten more chakras that exist purely at an auric level and do not descend to the physical body. They are considered to be above the Crown chakra above the level of the mental body. I first came across these in a wonderful little book by Colin Bloy called *I'm Just Going Down to the Pub to Do a Few Miracles*. This very tongue-in-cheek title belies its true message. The "outermost" of these auric chakras is called the "cup" or "chalice" chakra and is supposed to be several feet above the head. If you are interested in this very esoteric aspect of the chakras, please explore this in the book mentioned or in another tome. My book will not discuss healing at this level, since this type of knowledge could easily distract the budding hands-off practitioner.

TREATING THE AURIC REFLECTED CHAKRAS

The treatment of the auric reflected chakras was mentioned in Chapter 4, and this discipline may be performed using off-body techniques. The reflexologist can do several different things within the aura that would benefit to the patient.

Using KID 1

You will now be aware of the importance of this marvelous point (Foot chakra) in its effect on the rest of the body and in relaxation in particular. Instead of keeping the finger on the points, try to take the fingers into the etheric for some time. You will find that there is much more "power" underneath the fingertips than when using touch. What is more, when you start by touching KID 1 and you gently take your fingers into the etheric KID 1, the patient will insist that your fingers are still in contact with them!

Massaging the Aura

The technique of massaging the aura may be performed at the outset of the treatment session or during it. It is performed with the hands sweeping approximately one inch above the feet in a similar way to performing metamorphic technique. As your hands are massaging the aura around the feet, they will "pick up" the nuances of changes in the energy field, very similar to when this is performed on the body. When some "tingling," "spiking," or "shimmering" is felt, that is the region that needs to be treated later in the session. The emanation may be coming from one of the reflected chakras or from a reflected area.

Balancing the Auric Chakra Reflexes

Balancing the reflected chakras in the aura is exactly the same as balancing with your fingers on the skin. The same procedure of balancing left foot to right foot and then balancing top to bottom is performed, with the exception that the fingers are slightly off body. This technique is, obviously, slightly more difficult, and you will need to keep the hands and fingers very still (make sure that your forearms are very well supported on the couch). This technique is one of my favorites, and it is always a big hit when I teach it at workshops.

Treating the Auric Chakra Reflexes

In treating the auric chakra reflexes, once again there is no difference between this approach and the hands-on approach in the "batting order" required. Some reflexologists that I have taught over the years now only use this technique and tell me that they would never return to the hands-on approach.

I believe that with this book I have broken new ground in the field of energy medicine, and I hope that the average therapist will now undertake his or her own discipline in a new way. There is much more to know about the chakras that is outside the scope of this book. Chakras may be affected by sound, music, color, crystals, gemstones, herbs, Bach flower remedies, homeopathic medicines, tissue salts, meditation, hypnotherapy, radionics, radiesthesia, yoga, tai chi, and chi gong. Information on these topics and other aspects of the chakras such as astro-archeology, Ley lines (alignment of sacred sights), and the chakra energies of the earth can be found in other publications.

I love to receive feedback, queries, and general comments. Please go to my website, at www.johncrossclinics.com, for more details about my practice. You will also find information about how to order my full-color poster, "Healing with the Chakra Energy System," that is now in its eleventh year and fourth reprint. Thank you for reading this book, and the best of good luck to you all.

— YOU CAN BE WHATEVER YOU WANT TO BE —

*There is inside of you all of the potential to be whatever you want
     to be—*
All of the energy to do whatever you want to do.
Imagine yourself as you would like to be,
Doing what you want to do,
And every day, take one step toward your dream.
And although at times it may seem too difficult to continue,
Hold on to your dream.
*One morning you will awake to find that you are the person you
     dreamed of, doing what you wanted to do—*
Simply because you had the courage to believe in the potential
And to hold on to your dream.

Donna Levine

REFERENCES

Academy of Traditional Chinese Medicine. *An Outline of Chinese Acupuncture.* Beijing: Foreign Language Press, 1975.

Bartlett, S. *Auras—and How to Read Them.* London: Collins and Brown, 2000.

Bloy, C. *I'm Just Going Down to the Pub to Do a Few Miracles.* Devon, Eng.: Fountain International, 1990.

Brennan, B. A. *Hands of Light: A Guide to Healing Through the Human Energy Field.* New York: Bantam, 1987.

Charman, R. A., ed. *Complementary Therapies for Physical Therapists,* Oxford, Eng.: Butterworth Heinemann, 2000.

Coghill, R. *The Book of Magnetic Healing.* London: Gaia Books, 2000.

Cross, J. R. "The Relationship of the Chakra Energy System and Acupuncture." PhD diss. British College of Acupuncture, 1986.

———. *Acupressure: Clinical Applications in Musculo-Skeletal Conditions.* Oxford, Eng.: Butterworth Heinemann,, 2000.

———. *Acupressure and Reflextherapy in Medical Conditions,* Oxford, Eng.: Butterworth Heinemann, 2001.

———. "Avenues of Healing." *Newsletter of the Association of Chartered Physiotherapists in Energy Medicine* (2003): 5–9.

Ebner, M. *Connective Tissue Massage: Theory and Therapeutic Application.* Edinburgh: E. and S. Livingstone, 1962.

Gerber, R. *Vibrational Medicine: New Choices for Healing Ourselves.* Rochester, VT: Bear and Company, 1988.

———. *Vibrational Medicine for the 21st Century.* London: Piatkus, 2000.

Leadbeater, C. W. *The Chakras.* 1927. Reprint, Wheaton, IL: Theosophical Publishing House, 1982.

———. *The Inner Life.* 1958. Reprint, Wheaton, IL: Theosophical Publishing House, 1982.

Maitland, G. D. *Vertebral Manipulation,* 5th ed. London: Butterworth's, 1986.

McNaught, A., and R. Callander. *Illustrated Physiology.* London: E and S Livingstone, 1965.

Maxwell Cade, C. *The Awakened Mind.* 1979. Reprint, London: Element Books, 1996.

Motoyama, H. *Theories of the Chakras: Bridge to Higher Consciousness.* Theosophical Publishing House, 1988.

Shapiro, D. *Your Body Speaks Your Mind.* London: Piatkus, 1996.

Sills, F. *The Polarity Process.* Berkeley: North Atlantic Books, 2002.

Smith, C. W. *Energy Medicine and Measurement* and *Molecules, Memory and Communication.* Lecture, given to the Association of Chartered Physiotherapists in Energy Medicine (ACPEM), West Yorkshire, England, September 29, 2001. Copies available from Richard Harries, MCSP, conference secretary, 60 Rishworth Mill, Mill Lane, Rishworth, Sowerby Bridge, West Yorkshire HX6 4RZ.

Stormer, C. *Reflexology: The Definitive Guide.* London: Hodder and Stoughton, 1995.

———. *Language of the Feet.* London: Hodder and Stoughton, 1995.

Tansley, D. V. *Radionics and the Subtle Anatomy of Man.* Cambridge, Eng: C. W. Daniel, 1972.

———. *Subtle Body: Essence and Shadow.* Cambridge, Eng: C.W. Daniel, 1977.

———. *Chakras: Rays and Radionics.* C. W. Daniel, 1984.

Thie, J. F. *Touch for Health: A New Approach to Restoring Our Natural Energies.* Santa Monica, CA: De Vorss, 1979.

Walther, D. S. *Applied Kinesiology: The Advanced Approach in Chiropractic.* Pueblo, CO: Systems DC, 1976.

Williams, T. *Complete Chinese Medicine: A Comprehensive System for Health and Fitness.* Bath, Eng.: Element Books, 1996.

Zong-Xiang, Z. "Research Advances in the Electrical Specificity of Meridians and Acupuncture Points." *American Journal of Acupuncture* 9, no. 3 (1981): 203–16.

INDEX

Therapists, comfort for, 174–77
Thie, John, 124
Third eye, 63–64
Thoracic pain, 104
Thought forms, 15, 37–38
Throat
  conditions, 108
  sore, 70, 80
Throat chakra
  associations of, 68–69
  autonomic nervous system and, 56
  clairvoyant's view of, Color Plate 6
  color and, 59
  congested, 22
  emotions and, 55
  food allergies and, 33
  frequency range of, 39, 40
  function of, 67–68, 70
  Key point for, 53
  Large Intestine and Lung meridians and, 52
  position of, 44, 67
  reflexology treatment for, 223–25
  rotating vertices of, 58
  Sanskrit term for, 46
  sound and, 59
  spiritual connotation of, 55
  structure of, 20
  symbol for, 46
  symptomatology of, 70, 261
  thyroid and parathyroid glands and, 49
Thymus gland, 49
Thyroid gland, 49, 100
Tinnitus, 61, 104

TMJ syndrome, 66
Toes, holding, 206
Tonsillitis, 70, 91
Torticolis, 104
Traditional Chinese Medicine (TCM), 89, 111
Transplant surgery, 281
Traumas, 34–35
Triple Energizer meridian, 52
Tsubo. *See* Acupoints
Tubercular miasm, 32
Tumors
  benign, 73, 108
  breast, 91
  cancerous, 76

U
Ulcers, 32
  gravitational, 85, 91
  stomach, 76
Uncoordination, 22–23
Universal reflexology, 197
Unwinding, 140–41, 160–61

V
Varicosities, 73, 108
Vault hold, 250–52
Vertical reflextherapy, 197
Vertigo, 61, 66, 108
Vibrational Medicine (Gerber), 23, 36
Vibrational rates, 59
Viruses, 35, 91
Vital force, 40–42
  definition of, 11, 36
  manipulation of, 12
  names for, 11

Vitality, low, 80
Vomiting, 98
Vortices, rotating, 56–58, 275

W
Walther, David, 124
Water retention, 108
Worry, 66, 76, 108
Wrist joint, 145–46

Y
Yang imbalance, 44, 206
Yin imbalance, 44, 206
Your Body Speaks Your Mind
     (Shapiro), 266–67

Z
Zone therapy, 195, 197